Mother of
Methadone

Mother of Methadone

A DOCTOR'S QUEST, A FORGOTTEN HISTORY, AND A MODERN-DAY CRISIS

MELODY GLENN, MD

BEACON PRESS, BOSTON

BEACON PRESS
24 Farnsworth Street
Boston, Massachusetts
www.beacon.org

Beacon Press books
are published under the auspices of
the Unitarian Universalist Association of Congregations.

28 27 26 25   8 7 6 5 4 3 2 1

This book is printed on acid-free paper that meets the uncoated paper
ANSI/NISO specifications for permanence as revised in 1992.

Text design and composition by Kim Arney

Excerpts from the oral history interview between Dr. David Courtwright
and Dr. Marie Nyswander on June 22, 1981, held at
Columbia University, are printed here with permission.

*Library of Congress Cataloging-in-Publication
Data is available for this title.*
ISBN: 978-0-8070-1776-0; e-book: 978-0-8070-1775-3;
audiobook: 978-0-8070-2090-6

The authorized representative in the EU for product safety and
compliance is Easy Access System Europe 16879218, Mustamäe tee 50,
10621 Tallinn, Estonia: http://beacon.org/eu-contact

It all started with a question.

—DR. MARIE NYSWANDER

CONTENTS

AUTHOR'S NOTE

There is consensus that person-first language should be used when writing about someone with addiction, just as when writing about people with any other health condition, in order to reduce stigma and highlight that people are only secondarily defined by whatever illnesses plague them. This means that instead of saying "addict," one should use the terms "person with opioid use disorder," "person with chaotic drug use," or "people who use drugs" (PWUD). When working with patients, writing academic papers, or giving presentations to healthcare providers, I prefer the term "PWUD."

However, I worried that using this acronym too frequently in this book would pull readers out of the emotional story, especially in the context of historical periods when this acronym did not exist, so I occasionally use the word "addict" instead. Additionally, many people in recovery or who use drugs do not use person-first language, frequently using terms such as "addict," "clean," and "dirty." When I included such dialogue in the text, I tried to stay true to their original language. However, it is one thing for PWUD to decide to use these terms, and another entirely for clinicians. Healthcare providers should instead strive for person-first language.

This book blends memoir, history, and speculative nonfiction. As in most memoirs, the scenes taken from my own life are subject to the limitations of memory and perspective. For example, few of the conversations are verbatim transcripts. In cases of conflicting accounts, I often privileged my own version of events over others' recollections. To protect others' identities, especially those of patients, some names have been changed, and there are a few composite characters.

As there are absences in the archival record and many of the book's primary characters are no longer living, I often practiced "critical fabulation," a technique coined by Saidiya Hartman to narratively bridge the gaps with informed speculation. Speculative scenes are marked as such with phrases like "I imagined," "perhaps," and "maybe." I wrote them based on the best available evidence from primary source material. Unless quotes are marked as coming from interviews or articles, they are fictitious. For example, most of the scenes and corresponding dialogue from chapter 4 ("Narco") and the beginning of chapters 10 ("Zenith") and 11 ("The Fall") are imagined. Facts from research papers are cited as such.

The naming conventions used in this book differ from most academic texts in that I do not always refer to people by their last names, as I want to foster a sense of closeness with the book's main characters. However, referring to female physicians by their first name instead of their title and last name risks undermining their authority in healthcare. To strike a balance, I tended to use first names when the narrative calls for more intimacy and last names in more formal situations.

CHAPTER 1

The Clinic

2020

When I first neared the nondescript two-story building, I wasn't sure I was in the right place. There was no sign labeling what lay behind the drab stucco walls, and the windows were too few and too small to catch a glimpse. The clinic itself seemed ashamed of its own existence, or perhaps just worried about what the neighbors would think. The parking lot was surrounded by barbed wire and patrolled by a police officer. In the corner, just behind a tall, iron gate, a group of patients gathered. In the center an older woman lay on the pebbled ground, talking loudly in a scratchy voice between drags from her cigarette. A man wearing stained jeans and holding an extra-large Circle K cup stood beside a younger woman in flannel pajamas and chunky black slides. The officer had also noticed this congregation and was walking toward them; according to a posted sign, no loitering was allowed on the premises. I guided my bicycle to the rack behind them, a little worried whether it would still be there when I returned.

It was January 2020, and I was applying to work part-time as a physician at a methadone clinic. Primarily an emergency room doctor, I had become increasingly interested in addiction medicine over the past few years. To gain credibility—something I was always chasing as a young woman in medicine—I decided to pursue board certification in the field. This meant that I needed to work at least five hundred clinical hours in addiction, and in Tucson the only place looking for help was a methadone clinic. I had never imagined myself working somewhere like this; methadone clinics weren't exactly seen as desirable. Nobody in my medical school aspired to work at one, nor was it presented as a career goal that we might strive for. But here I was, in a nice dress and leather boots, with freshly washed hair, ready for my interview.

Swinging open the tinted glass door, I entered the buzz of the crowded waiting room. A line of patients formed to my right, waiting to get their daily doses. The air smelled of stale cigarettes and cherry cough syrup, the flavor added to the liquid methadone. Many of the patients had sunburned shoulders, and a few had cheap, thin rollerbags that they dragged alongside them—signs of housing insecurity.

To my left was a sea of vinyl chairs filled with patients waiting to see therapists, clinicians, or lab techs. Several times a year, patients were randomly selected to give a urine sample to determine whether they were still using drugs. They peed into cups held over toilets with silver handles taped in place to remind them of the rules, which were printed on a piece of paper, highlighted in yellow, and tacked to the rear wall—no flushing the toilet or running the faucet—even though there was no sink inside the small bathroom itself. There was also no lock on the door. The freshness of the sample was verified by a flimsy thermometer attached to the cup. The printed rules also detailed what happened if someone couldn't pee within three minutes: if they decided to leave the clinic instead of waiting in the lobby and trying again, a staff member would watch them urinate when they next returned. If my doctor asked me to follow such condescending, punitive rules, I would be outraged. I would demand to see their policies, argue with the staff, or storm out. But if you wanted methadone, there was no choice but to comply.

One of the employees noticed me standing awkwardly in the entryway. "Can I help you?" he asked.

"I have an appointment with Dr. Oñate." The words rushed out of my mouth a little too quickly.

"Okay, stand in line here." He pointed to a line forming at the front desk, a layer of bulletproof plexiglass separating the clerks from the patients.

"But I'm not a . . ." I swallowed the final word of this sentence, *patient*, realizing how rude I appeared, how quick I was to set myself apart from those around me. "I'm here to interview for a part-time position."

He smiled. I wasn't telling him anything he didn't know. "He's on his way; we are texting him. You can have a seat." I sat down across from two women chatting, one with her young son, who was singing quietly and swaying his head back and forth. The other woman was in the middle of explaining how she was trying to get her kids back. After I started working here, I'd learn this was common. Many of my patients, especially the women, had open cases with the Department of Child Services (DCS), their kids now in foster care or living with relatives. How different than my own experience, in which my soon-to-be-one-year-old was currently in the loving arms of our full-time nanny.

An older man with salt-and-pepper hair and tanned skin walked through the side door. "Hi, I'm Larry. Sorry I'm late." He extended his hand to shake mine. This was Dr. Oñate, the medical director of the clinic. "We had a bit of a commotion this morning—maybe you saw it outside as you arrived. There was a woman selling outside, which is a big no-no around here." He shook his head. "We contract with TPD—Tucson Police Department—to provide our security, and they arrested her. It's usually much calmer than that." He smiled. I followed him as he badged us out of the waiting room and opened a locked door, his cowboy boots clicking across the linoleum floor.

First, we visited the "dosing room," where more plexiglass separated the staff from the patients. The nurses sat along a long counter, each manning a dispensing machine. Cheerfully, they paused to wave and introduce themselves, the jovial atmosphere seemingly at odds with the harsh security measures.

Dr. Oñate and I stood next to one of the nurses while a man and his small child approached her window. Gasping for breath, the man exclaimed, "Our car just broke down, and I had to get it jumped." He had made it just in time—"dosing hours" were observed strictly, 5 to 11 a.m. and 1 to 5 p.m. If a patient came outside those times, they would be turned away, no matter the reason. And if they missed more than two days in a row, their dose would be halved into an effectively useless amount. It would take days, if not weeks, to again reach a therapeutic level. Regulations did not make recovery easy. During the hour "lunch break," the nurses meticulously tallied the amount of methadone dispensed during the morning. If even a single drop was unaccounted for, the DEA could shut the whole place down.

As the man on the other side of the window spoke, the nurse clicked through a series of questions about his appearance, pupil size, and speech; she had to document that he wasn't high. She then clicked the dispense button, and the machine released a few milliliters of red liquid into the plastic cup below. The man poured some water into the liquid, swirled it around, threw his head back, and tossed the concoction into his mouth. He waved goodbye as he walked away, his smiling son's hand clasped tightly in his own.

"Why did he add the water to the cup?" I asked.

The nurse, behind her thick-framed, black glasses, answered. "To get all the methadone. Sometimes five to ten milligrams are left behind on the sides of the cup."

I nodded, not yet understanding that the difference between fifty and sixty milligrams could cause the sweats, chills, and nausea of withdrawal.

She continued: "This was the first job I took after nursing school, and I can't imagine doing anything else." She paused. "I wanted to see what my husband goes through. Just last week, we got a cake and celebrated ten years sober." She smiled. "For the people who want to quit and turn their lives around, there is nothing like this. Methadone really works."

Initially synthesized in the 1930s, methadone was developed in an attempt to find a long-lasting, nonaddictive pain medication. Although chemists are still searching for that panacea, we found a role for methadone in daily maintenance therapy. Itself an opioid, it is still habit-forming and can cause overdose if taken in excessive amounts, but, by the numbers, it is much safer than heroin or fentanyl. Unlike street drugs, its manufacture is regulated, so users know exactly what they are getting and in what amount. Its pharmacology is also slightly different, allowing for long-term stability instead of the extreme highs and lows associated with short-acting fentanyl and heroin. And because it is legal, it reduces the risky behaviors and negative consequences associated with addiction.

This is not to say that methadone maintenance is perfect. If patients miss a few days of methadone, they go into the same bone-crushing withdrawal that they did back when they couldn't find any dope. It is still an opioid. And, so, many recovery organizations preach that a drug is a drug, that methadone is no different than heroin. To me, it is easy to poke holes in this claim.

Although related, dependence and addiction are different. Dependence means that someone has tolerance to and withdrawal from a medication or substance they take daily—like getting a caffeine headache when you miss your morning cup of coffee—whereas addiction, or a substance use disorder, is a medical condition with specific diagnostic criteria defined by the *Diagnostic and Statistical Manual of Mental Disorders*, including: taking in larger amounts and for longer than intended, wanting to cut down or quit but not being able to, spending a lot of time obtaining the substance, craving or experiencing a strong desire to use, being unable to carry out major obligations due to the substance, and continuing to use despite the harms it causes. Most people taking methadone do have dependence, yet very few are addicted. But the simplest rebuttal is an analogy offered frequently by Dr. Marie Nyswander, one first attributed to the jazz musician Billie Holiday: Did we tell people with diabetes to stop using insulin because their body needed it? Of course not. From a medical standpoint, methadone is no different.

It was with pride that Dr. Oñate continued his tour of the clinic's facilities, each step peeling back the harsh veneer of my first impression. He showed me the spacious room where tai chi classes were offered, a play area for the patients' children, and quiet suites for families who needed to stay the night.

"We even have acupuncture," he boasted, lifting his bushy eyebrows for emphasis. I found it hard to believe that the clinic's rules and enforcement came from him, someone whom I imagined listened to community radio on the weekends while drinking a cup of tea in a garden overgrown with tendrils of cat's claw and shaded by leafy ironwood trees. As I would come to learn, these harsh standards came from the DEA, Substance Abuse and Mental Health Services Administration (SAMHSA), and Congress—the rules a bureaucratically confusing hodgepodge cobbled together throughout the decades in a way that seemed to take little interest in the lived experience of the people they were intended to help.

From the second-floor "balcony," a thin and unadorned precipice of concrete that ran along the length of the building, I could better see the surrounding neighborhood. The southern edge of the parking lot abutted several trailers, and the western edge was marked by coiled barbed wire running alongside an iron fence. But it was with pride that Dr. Oñate talked about the surrounding community.

"We try really hard to show that we are good neighbors." Every week, a group of patients—or, as the clinic referred to them, "members"—circled the nearby streets to pick up the litter and trash strewn by the dry desert winds.

I lifted an eyebrow. Why did they try so hard to garner approval? Other medical clinics didn't do that. And it wasn't like this clinic was in the middle of a perfectly manicured neighborhood; the building next door had broken windows patched by black plastic bags fluttering in the breeze, and the closest businesses were a liquor store and a vape shop. It certainly didn't look like my neighborhood: historic adobe houses painted in pastel, abundant shade trees, and beautifully xeriscaped yards. In this part of town, there were no college kids jogging, new parents pushing strollers, or stately professors cycling by. In fact, I didn't see anybody outside the clinic's immediate periphery.

Dr. Oñate continued: "Another clinic in town doesn't try so hard to integrate itself into the community, and they've had problems." A smooth calmness metered his speech. "Instead of taking the time to establish relationships, or to build something of quality, they are focusing on rapid expansion."

Although I nodded in agreement, I wondered how that was a problem. Fentanyl was now the leading cause of death in young adults and one of the top contenders among all other age groups. With so many more people needing access to addiction treatment, expansion seemed like exactly what was needed to combat the current crisis.

"And so now," he explained, "one of the communities in which they built a new clinic is trying to shut them down. They don't want *those kinds of people* in the neighborhood."

Opposition to one clinic could easily snowball and threaten them all: if a clinic didn't do a good enough job of looking presentable, if it seemed too sketchy or derelict, neighbors might start to distrust all methadone clinics, soon demanding that politicians develop stricter zoning regulations to further curtail their development. Ideally, the solution would be to convince the public that treating addiction was good and worthwhile. But that was too gargantuan a task for a single clinic to take on, so, instead, they had to play the defensive, to look nice. Soon, I would learn that this tension between access and quality stretched all the way back to methadone's inception.

After Dr. Oñate finished his tour, we returned to his office to discuss the details. Although I had prepared for the rigorous back-and-forth of an interview, the job was mine if I wanted it.

Dr. Oñate leaned back in his swivel chair, tapping his fingertips together in front of his chest and staring toward the ceiling before his eyes refocused on mine. "Now, I know that most of your experience is with buprenorphine, but I really hope you will use your time here to learn about methadone, to realize that it is the better option for a lot of our patients."

I laughed awkwardly and averted my gaze. He had seen right through me. Although methadone and buprenorphine, often referred to by its trade name Suboxone or the abbreviated "bupe," are both types of medications for opioid use disorder (MOUD), I had always believed bupe the preferential option.

Imagine zooming in on a large, squishy brain, right up to the cellular level. Stuck into one of the neurons is a stick topped with a cup—the mu opioid receptor—and floating toward it is a ball—a molecule of fentanyl. When the two meet, the brain's frequencies slow. Alertness flickers off, causing a peaceful sense of sleep. Pain dulls, both that inflicted by a sharp kick to the shins or from the deeper pains of psychological trauma. Unfortunately, the lungs also relax to the brink of failure, serenely ignoring the body's hunger for oxygen. If too many of the cups fill with fentanyl, the body's workings come to a grinding halt, a phenomenon better known as "overdose."

Methadone, just like heroin, just like oxycodone, just like fentanyl, is a full opioid agonist. The more you take, the more euphoria, sedation, and respiratory depression. Although buprenorphine is also a ball that fits into the cup of the mu receptor, it is a partial agonist, meaning its downstream effects are much less noticeable and intense. It is like using a dimmer switch to turn down a light's glare. Even if someone takes a dose ten times higher than what is prescribed, nothing much happens, at least for patients who regularly take opioids. They are still awake, conversant, and breathing. There is a ceiling to buprenorphine's effects.

Because of the lesser risk, buprenorphine is much less regulated than methadone. I can write a prescription for buprenorphine to be picked up at any pharmacy, whereas patients who want methadone must come every day to a federally recognized clinic and drink their medication under a nurse's watchful eye. In fact, methadone is one of the most regulated medications in America. God forbid a patient has to leave town, as they can't simply get a few days' worth of methadone to take with them. Instead, they must find a clinic in whatever city they are visiting—if there even is one—get permission from their home clinic to apply for guest dosing, and fax over a bunch of paperwork. Although recent regulation changes have made it slightly easier to get "take-homes," the poison is still more accessible than the treatment.[1]

And, thus, I unapologetically preferred buprenorphine over methadone, as did the small, rising wave of emergency medicine physicians who were prescribing MOUD. Whereas I had started countless patients on buprenorphine and had educated other providers how to do the same, I had never started a patient on methadone.

Even here at a methadone clinic, I planned to rarely use it, instead offering bupe as the first-line option. But, as Dr. Oñate continued his spiel about medicine's favoritism of bupe over methadone, I began to question myself. Was my preference for buprenorphine simply part of a larger trend, one rooted in stigma instead of science? A stigma I thought I had long left behind? As the glass door of the clinic closed behind me, scarlet shame unfurled across my cheeks as I remembered how I once treated people who used drugs.

2015

"Can you please go see room thirteen? He's being a real pain in the ass." The nurse glared and flipped her platinum blonde hair behind her shoulders. Nobody had time for bullshit on a night shift. I squinted under the fluorescent lights of the "doc box," the square room in the middle of the emergency department where the residents and supervising attending physicians clicked through labs and typed patient notes. House music pulsed from a speaker propped on a cluttered shelf overhead—the only way to trick our bodies that 3 a.m. was a good time to be awake. It was 2015, and I was a junior emergency medicine resident at the county hospital in Phoenix. Even though it was 110 degrees outside, in here I wore a jacket to insulate against the subarctic air conditioning.

I blinked to clear the fatigue from my dry eyes. I was in the middle of a month of night shifts, working from 10 p.m. to 8 a.m., Sunday to Thursday. Even if I got sick, I was still expected to show up. Such was residency. Once, when my body shook with fever and swallowing my own spit felt like shards of glass, I checked in an hour before my shift so I could at least get a throat swab and throw down some antibiotics. It was not unheard of for doctors to work with IVs threaded into their forearms so they could medicate between seeing patients. When the $500 bill came a few weeks later, I regretted my decision. Although I was earning more than I ever had—a little less than $50,000 a year—I wasn't exactly in a position to throw away money for a penicillin prescription, not with my student loans and their 6 percent interest. And if the sleep deprivation, lack of sick leave, and bullying from the nurses and senior residents were not enough, there also was the constant terror that I would make a fatal mistake. And so, as residency dragged on, I found it harder and harder to feel much empathy for some of my patients. Although I knew that was wrong, I just didn't have anything left to give.

The nurse leaned against the wall, refusing to leave until one of us claimed the patient in room thirteen, and stared straight at me. Or was that a glare? Although she helped and flirted with the male residents, she mainly complained about the women. And because I knew she would make the rest of my shift a living hell if I pissed her off, I stood and plucked the plastic clipboard from the wall rack. According to the triage sheet, he had checked in for lower back pain and claimed to be allergic to all our first- and even our second-line options for pain control: acetaminophen, ibuprofen, Toradol, morphine, oxycodone. I was sure he would ask for Dilaudid, one of the strongest opioids we had. In a study in which people who used heroin received either a shot of Dilaudid or heroin, they couldn't tell the difference. I rolled my eyes as I asked the nurse, "He's a pain seeker, huh?" It was something we saw a lot back then, back before cheap fentanyl flooded the streets.

She nodded in agreement before pivoting and disappearing down the hallway.

I slid open the glass doors to his room. He was writhing around on the narrow stretcher, his long, lanky frame curled into a Z. When he saw me from the corner of his eye, he increased the volume of his moans to an unbearable holler. I was certain of it—he was here for drugs, willing to make up whatever complaint necessary to get them. But, of course, I couldn't just write that in his medical record. First, I would have to prove that there was nothing wrong with him. Only then could I discharge him and wash my hands of this hassle.

Patients commonly came to the ED for low back strain caused by bending over or lifting something a little too heavy. Nothing dangerous. Unfortunately, there were a handful of rare conditions that looked the same but were much more serious: an abscess next to the spinal cord, cancer eating away at the vertebrae, or a tear shedding the aorta's sinewy wall. It was up to us ED docs to determine if a patient's symptoms were caused by a life-threatening condition or just everyday wear and tear, and it wasn't always so easy to tell the difference.

I sat down on the black stool next to him and crossed my arms. "Do you have difficulty urinating?" I interrogated.

"Yes," he answered, not missing a beat.

I continued right on to the next question, trying to keep my voice calm. I wanted to appear indifferent. I did not want my face to betray the rage building inside me. I also did not want him to think I actually believed him—I was no fool. "Do you have decreased sensation between your thighs?"

"Yes."

I sighed, but I doubted that he noticed; he was too busy squeezing his eyes shut and fake crying. He was going to make this difficult. Well seasoned at this game, he knew all the "right" answers, the ones that would extend his visit and lead to the maximum number of Dilaudid shots. Perhaps he visited a different ED each night—there were certainly plenty of people like that here in Phoenix. He probably took an ambulance, too, so he didn't have to pay any money up front for the ride. Looking back now, I am ashamed of my cruel cynicism. But back then, I heard remarks like this so often they seemed normal. And what else is residency but an indoctrination into the hidden curriculum of medicine?

Of course, there was the chance I could be wrong, and the penalty for error would be this man's life. And if he injected drugs like I assumed, he was at even higher risk for invasive infections that could very well hide in the spine. Reusing needles meant that bacteria was injected directly into the bloodstream, where it spread quickly to every organ in the body. Even though I wanted to dismiss his answers, I knew I couldn't. But that didn't mean I had to like him.

My voice monotone, I continued: "Okay. We will need some blood, and maybe even some imaging."

He flung the coarse cotton blanket over his head, his curled toes the only part of his body still visible. "Doc," he said, his voice now muffled, "I'm really in a lot of pain. I can't answer any more questions until you give me Dilaudid."

I pursed my lips and marched toward the doc box to order his labs, peripheral IV, and Dilaudid. I hated to give in to his demands, especially when it involved giving an opioid that was almost equivalent to heroin. If there was one thing that my medical training had taught me about opioids, it was that doctors needed to limit our use of them. Time and time again, we were told that doctors' liberal prescribing of oxycodone was to blame for the current opioid epidemic, and that if we just limited the supply of drugs that we gave, nobody would become hooked. Later, I'd learn that this was just a repackaged version of a distorted claim probably as old as drugs themselves. Additionally, I had unknowingly bought into the stigma that people who want to keep using drugs didn't deserve our care.

I also didn't want to give him the high he was seeking—that wasn't why I was here. Something about it felt immoral, or maybe just unfair. I was the one working an overnight shift, my eyelids heavy, my body longing to lie down, and he wanted me to help him get high? But I saw no other way. If I wanted to rule out infection, I needed a sample of his blood to send to the lab. Without the Dilaudid, he would probably flail his arm as the nurse attempted to slide the sharp tip of the needle into his vein, potentially causing her hand to slip and stick her own finger.

On the tracking board, I saw that an ambulance had just brought a new patient to the resuscitation bay, and I hurried to meet them. It was not just the man in room thirteen whom I was responsible for. I arrived just as the Phoenix Fire medics were leaving, a blast of hot, dry air gusting through the double doors as they returned into the desert night. Even at these hours, the breeze felt oppressive.

The new patient was short and plump, her eyes rolling back into her head as she spoke. Never a good sign. A nurse and a tech quickly worked in seamless choreography to connect a tangle of wires from her chest to the monitor hanging in the corner overhead, insert IVs, and draw vials of maroon blood from her narrow veins. Once attached, the monitor wouldn't shut up, its loud alarm firing constantly from her abnormally low blood pressure and oxygen levels. I rolled the heavy ultrasound machine over to her bedside to visualize her heart and lungs upon its grayscale monitor. Was her blood pressure dangerously low because her heart wasn't pumping effectively? No. Were her lungs filled with fluid? No. So what was the cause? I requested antibiotics and fluids while I prepared to intubate and place a central line. There was no time to waste.

But before I could set up everything, the portable black phone in my back pocket began to ring and vibrate. The nurse on the other end said, "Hey, Doc, your patient in room thirteen won't let us stick him anymore until we give him more pain medication, and I'm having a hard time getting an IV."

As I looked at the dying woman in front of me, I spoke into the phone: "Were you at least able to get the blood for the lab?"

"No, he's a hard stick." Years of IV drug use often scarred the veins and the overlying skin, so I wasn't surprised by this.

The respiratory therapist was now strapping a plastic mask to the woman's face, a CPAP machine pushing air into her lungs before I attempted to place a breathing tube through her gaping mouth and into her trachea. Streams of air whooshed out the sides of the loose mask, but she didn't even notice, her eyelids now closed.

"I'll swing by his room and try, but I can't be there long," I told the nurse on the other end of the line. Here was a critically ill woman who needed my care, but, instead, I had to deal with this addict's antics. Although he would probably die within a few years from an overdose or the complications of injecting, I still did not see him as the high-acuity patient he was. But the faster I freed up his bed, the faster I could help the sick patients who sat waiting in the lobby, so I walked quickly to his room. The haze of early morning continued like this for hours, seesawing between him and the dozen other patients under my care.

When the results from his labs and MRI finally came back, it was exactly as I suspected—everything was perfectly normal. When I went to tell him, he already knew the jig was up. For the first time all night, he was now sitting quietly in bed, eating one of the dry turkey sandwiches that we kept in the patient fridge. Hot rage bubbled in my chest. I hated that he had wasted our time and money, that he had stolen it from others who I thought needed it more. I hated that he had bent me to his will. Even though I knew he was lying, my hands had been tied. I hated working with addicts—it always seemed to end like this.

But why? I had read the textbook, passed all the exams, and yet here I was, flailing. The only detail about addiction that I remembered from medical school was that Dr. Drew of MTV's *Loveline* gave us a one-hour lecture. Although I can't recall a single detail of the content, I do remember the glamour of a celebrity physician standing right there in front of us. I suppose this was the kind of thing that happened when you went to medical school in Los Angeles. And although my school wasn't exactly a beacon of light when it came to addiction—our dean's face later plastered across the front page of *The Los Angeles Times* under the headline "An Overdose, a Young Companion, Drug-Fueled Parties: The Secret Life of a USC Med School Dean"—most medical schools across the country similarly glossed over addiction.

The content taught during my emergency medicine residency wasn't much better, and, again, my experience wasn't an outlier. The only mention of opioid use disorder in my ten-pound textbook was a paltry two pages, mainly focused on when and how to reverse overdoses with naloxone in the ED.[2] Nowhere did it describe opioid use disorder as a chronic disease, nowhere did it explain how to diagnose it, and it certainly didn't mention that it had an effective treatment. Although the Food and Drug Administration (FDA) approved buprenorphine in 2002, I had never heard of it, and I didn't know much more about methadone. And there was definitely no mention of harm reduction, an approach that sought to reduce the harms associated with drug use and meet patients where they were. And, so, my patients and I held opposing stories of addiction and treatment, leaving little room for a shared narrative.

I also lacked lived experience with addiction, or so I thought. Although I was high for most of college, it was easy for me to step away. I didn't really drink until medical school, an institution where binge drinking was normalized. During one party, an ambulance carried away a friend of mine because he drank too much. Another friend frequently blacked out on the weekends. Yet nobody talked about it. Neither did my family, really. I had heard hushed stories about my late grandfather's problematic use of morphine, but always in the context of being weak. Never mentioned was the trauma that increased his risk of addiction: he was born Jewish in 1915 Poland, lost most of his family, fought in the war, and aspired to assimilation in America. In my life, it was easy to ignore addiction, to see it as a problem that happened to someone else.

And, from a medical perspective, I had learned that addiction was a hopeless condition that lacked an effective treatment, rendering me powerless under its gaze. As the medical profession often does with conditions it does not understand, we looked away. Instead of facing the possibility that we might not know everything, we blamed the patients. We treated users with disdain and called them "drug seekers." We thought they were manipulative liars, manufacturing medical complaints that they hoped might result in a prescription for painkillers.

Although the opioid epidemic was all over the news, effective treatment had not made its way into most clinics or hospitals. Out of nearly one million doctors in the United States, less than six hundred identified themselves as addiction specialists in 2012.[3] That might be okay if doctors from other specialties knew how to treat addiction, but they didn't. Instead, doctors focused on treating the secondary, more costly complications that resulted from chronic use—liver cirrhosis, HIV, endocarditis, cellulitis, hepatitis C, cancer, heart disease, overdose—allowing the underlying addiction to continue unchecked. Today's shortage of physicians trained to treat addiction means that only 10 percent of the forty million Americans with addiction receive any formal treatment at all, and, when they do, it is rarely based on evidence. Later, I'd learn that this negligence was not accidental, nor was it new; we were simply following a precedent set over a century ago.

Because medical providers have neglected addiction for so long, a separate, nonscientific, and poorly regulated network of addiction care has developed. Patients face a confusing patchwork of treatment options with wildly different approaches. There are expensive residential treatments with little data to justify their cost, tough-love, style rehabs, work-based communities, medical detox facilities, and

12-step programs, just to name a few. A 2012 report by Columbia University compared the state of addiction medicine today to that of general medicine practiced in the early 1900s, both overrun by a preponderance of quacks selling snake oil.[4] Most of the people providing addiction care have received little, if any, formal training, and thus many still think of addiction as a moral or spiritual failing. The public has a similar view, with about one-third believing that addiction reflects a lack of self-control or willpower.

But the science is clear—addiction is a disease. Over the last half century, scientists have identified which parts of the brain are involved in aberrant behaviors: the basal ganglia with euphoria, the amygdala with withdrawal, and the prefrontal cortex with anticipation for more.[5] Furthermore, the continued use of drugs actually alters the structure and function of the brain, making people want to use even more, despite negative consequences.[6] This means that harsh penalties and lengthy jail time will not work as effective deterrents, although many lawmakers believe they will. Incarceration is not treatment.

In the addiction medicine textbook from which I now teach, there is a grayscale snapshot of two brains.[7] One is from a healthy person, and one is from a person with addiction. The contrast between the two is glaringly obvious. The healthy brain glows a bright white, its active neurons quickly zipping messages back and forth. In contrast, the diseased brain is a dull gray, the neurons effectively offline or even dead. It looks just like an injured heart starved of oxygen, one whose muscles died after a massive attack.

That being said, not everyone who uses drugs becomes addicted, and the simple use of an illicit or mind-altering substance does not mean that someone has a disorder; it is only when that use causes problems in a person's life that we become concerned.[8] Recently, scientists have even pinpointed specific genes that make someone more or less likely to be addicted—more evidence that addiction is linked to concrete pathology in the brain.[9] Yet genes alone aren't enough, as not everyone with at-risk genetics develops a problem. Trauma, especially in childhood, also seems to play a large role. One famous study suggested that two-thirds of problematic drug use could be attributed to adverse childhood experiences such as abuse, neglect, or growing up in a household with substance abuse, incarceration, or mental illness.[10]

Despite the advent of sophisticated imaging technology and advanced methods that allow us to visualize individual genes, scientists still don't fully understand addiction. We have theories about who is at risk and who might get better, but no two patients are exactly alike. This could also be said about many other diseases, such as cancer, chronic pain, or even COVID. That is the thing about science: we are constantly learning new information that shifts existing theories. The more I learn about medicine, the more I learn how little is absolute.

There is even a growing critique of the "addiction as disease" framework. Although it was supposed to reduce the stigma faced by PWUD and increase access to treatment, for many people this has not been the case. The disease model does not adequately address the societal causes of addiction, such as the trauma caused by inequity and racism, instead implying that there is something inherently pathologic about the brains of people who use drugs and become dependent. Although I agree with these statements, I do not think they are antithetical to the concept of addiction as a disease. I also think that arguing over semantics distracts from issues that matter more: stigma, onerous policy, and over a century of criminalizing addiction and its treatment.

2020

When I returned home from my interview at the methadone clinic, I began my search for an origin story, suspecting that my seemingly personal unease around methadone was actually a reflection of something much bigger. When did methadone treatment first come onto the scene? How was it received? On the front page of an old *JAMA* article commemorating the forty-year anniversary of methadone maintenance, a black-and-white photo of a female physician caused me to pause, to look closer.[11] She was about sixty or seventy, joy radiating from her eyes. Perhaps this was what it looked like to be proud of your life's work. She was seated in a library, her bangs swept to one side, her hair cut short around her face. Bracelets adorned her slim wrists, and she was wearing a white button-down blouse tucked into a high-waisted skirt. A large pendant in the shape of a rounded cross hung from a chain around her neck. Her name was Dr. Marie Nyswander. Beside her stood a balding man with a closed-mouth grin and a long white coat—Dr. Vincent Dole. Together, they had developed methadone maintenance. Later, I would learn that they had also fallen in love while spending long hours together in the hospital, when she was in her late forties and he in his late fifties, and that he was her fourth husband and she his second wife, but this article only mentioned them as research partners.

The article focused on their landmark 1965 study in which they proved that daily methadone could treat heroin addiction, relieving cravings and allowing people with addiction to return to stable lives.[12] At the time, nobody else in the United States was researching or offering maintenance treatment for addiction, mainly because it was illegal to do so. Instead, treatments were abstinence based and predicated on the idea that addiction was a moral failure or evidence of psychopathy, and relapse rates teetered around 90 percent. But, with their study, Nyswander and Dole suggested that addiction was a medical disease for which they had a successful treatment. One addiction physician described their results as equally monumental as the discovery of the first antibiotic.[13]

Although methadone maintenance was lauded as the panacea to end opioid addiction forever, the opioid epidemic today is exponentially worse than anything Dr. Nyswander could have imagined. According to the Centers for Disease Control and Prevention, more than two million Americans have opioid use disorder, and fatal overdoses have surpassed motor vehicle collisions as the most frequent cause of accidental death.[14] In 2021, over one hundred thousand Americans died from overdose.[15] What had transpired between Marie's time and now? How did methadone fail? In the article, Dr. Mary Jeanne Kreek, an addiction physician who worked with Nyswander and Dole at Rockefeller University, offered an explanation that resonated completely with my own experience: "There is a stigma against addictions, addicts, and—sadly—treatment providers."

I peered into Marie's eyes, a sense of kinship building. At age thirty-four, I was an aspiring addiction physician looking for a role model, and Marie's story drew me in with her promise of a medical fairy tale about a pioneering, revolutionary physician who broke the rules on behalf of a group of patients whom mainstream society would prefer to ignore. On the surface, her story seemed equivalent to those portrayed by Hollywood in *And the Band Played On* and the *Dallas Buyers Club*, inspirational movies about the power of medicine to fight injustice. Yet it wasn't the medicine that really pulled viewers in, but a charismatic protagonist, usually a white male, who fought the system and led others toward a better future. Hope fluttered in my chest—had I finally discovered a version of this story with a female lead?

I had always craved a female boss or mentor in medicine, but they were hard to come by. It was only recently that women and men matriculated at equal rates into medical school, and women are still much less likely to be chairs, directors, or full professors. Of my residency's twenty or so faculty members, only two were women, and neither held a position of authority. In the community EDs where I later worked, all the directors and chairs were men. Although the men who had mentored me were wonderful, there were some things they would never understand. They would never have to pump breast milk while on a busy ER shift or feel the same pressure to choose between family or career. And leadership strategies that worked for them would not always have the same effect for me.

I saw Marie's life as a potential key to all my questions, and I began to unravel it like a detective. I searched far and wide for clues, turning to books, archival articles, and interviews. Who was she, professionally and personally? What could she teach me about the history of addiction treatment and today's related inability to stymie a worsening epidemic? About what it means to be a doctor facing the double stigma of treating addiction and being a woman? Why did I get the sense that I was fighting the same battles, with myself, my patients, and medicine at large, that Marie already fought more than fifty years ago?

———

Within a few days, I went to the library and checked out Marie's book, *The Drug Addict as a Patient*. I ordered her 1968 biography penned by Nat Hentoff, a staff writer at *The New Yorker*. I traced all the citations on her Wikipedia page. But everything I found told more or less the same abbreviated story, a series of dates and details that barely scratched the surface. They repeated the same anecdotes. There was the year she spent at the Lexington, Kentucky, Narcotic Farm because the US Navy did not have a uniform for women; the Christmas when she gave out morphine shots as presents to the incarcerated men; the clinic for jazz musicians that she cofounded; her various husbands.

They all painted her the same way—as a rebellious and infectiously captivating woman who was helping a group of people the rest of the world would rather forget. Why hadn't she become more of a sensation? Why had only one biography been written, and over fifty years ago? Why was I only now learning of her? Why weren't young healthcare workers holding her up as an icon?

Although the mythology of her hero narrative certainly entranced me, I also hoped her life would somehow illuminate an alternative path to the doctor-as-savior trope, a concept I had been wrestling with for years. Because I aspired to make the world a better place, I became a doctor, which meant that I did occasionally save people, yet I didn't want to be anybody's savior. Although this slight distinction made sense theoretically, in practice the margins were not so clear.

Fairly quickly, I came to the end of the materials I could easily find about Marie—obituaries, *New York Times* articles, Hentoff's biography, and her two books—but the more I learned about her, the more questions I had. I became obsessed with finding anyone from Marie's life who might still be alive. To gather more angles of Marie and arrange them into a fully fleshed out character, I wanted to speak to the people who knew her. But where to find them?

I began my search from my office at CODAC, the methadone clinic where I was now working one day a week. Since I was new, I did not yet have a panel of established patients to fill my schedule, and much of my time was spent waiting for new clients to walk in. I was not used to such downtime; I literally wore running shoes in the emergency department. Alone in an office, there was nobody to talk to. To fill the empty hours, I hunched over my computer desk and scoured the internet for clues about Marie.

Although most of Marie's colleagues were no longer alive—something to be expected when writing about someone born in 1919—a few were. I emailed Dr. Mary Jeanne Kreek, the young physician whom Marie and Vincent had involved in their early methadone research, and who currently directed Rockefeller University's Laboratory of the Biology of Addictive Diseases. Who better to share some insight into Marie's personality than someone who worked alongside her during the early days of their discovery and had been there when she and Vince were falling in love? But she did not respond. A few months later, I tried again. Still, no response.

Sometime later, I learned there was somewhat of a rivalry between Marie and Mary Jeanne, the latter believing she had been unfairly denied credit for her role in discovering methadone maintenance. She was just an intern when she joined their team; had Vince and Marie treated her poorly because of her low rank? Her gender? Perhaps Mary Jeanne would be the one to reveal some less favorable aspects of Marie's personality, providing an example of how *not* to be. When months passed with still no response, I assumed Mary Jeanne was tired of talking about Marie, of forever remaining under her shadow instead of allowed to shine in her own right. But when I came across her obituary in *The New York Times*, I realized there had been another reason for her silence. Time was running out.

As the months passed, my search for information seemed to be leading me in circles, repeating the same stories and dates. Hitting a roadblock, I began to doubt the entire project. This emotion only intensified as I became more and more pregnant with my second daughter, hormones casting a generalized anxiety that hummed constantly in the background. But I couldn't stop.

One night, my laptop resting upon the curve of my belly, I re-read one of the short biographies of Marie I'd found online. At that point I probably could have recited it from memory like one of my daughter's picture books, which were scattered around me in a post-bedtime mess I didn't have the energy to pick up.

Just for fun, I clicked on one of the hyperlinks that took me to the endnotes. Most of them referred to the same articles and books that I'd already read, some of them so many times that I could place on the page where they were in the corresponding text. But there was one entry that I swear hadn't been there before:

"Oral history interviews with Marie Nyswander (1981) and Vincent Dole (1982) are housed at the Columbia University Oral History Center."

I paused. Perhaps, instead of struggling to read handwritten letters on yellowing sheets scanned into PDFs, I could actually hear her voice, pick out new traces of her personality. Eyes nearly closed with fatigue, I scoured the website for Columbia's archives and requested the files. I had no sense of whether they would send them—perhaps they were limited to those within the walls of the ivory tower—but I hoped that my university-affiliated email might at least pique their interest. I slept a little better that night, I think. It felt like I'd at least done something.

A few days later, I was standing in front of a group of firefighters in Nogales, Arizona, a sleepy town split in half by the US-Mexico border, instructing them how to give out naloxone, the medication that reverses opioid overdoses, to community members at risk. As I paused to wipe the beads of sweat off my forehead from the after-noon heat, I suggested that everyone break for a few minutes before we moved on to discussing buprenorphine and methadone. Sitting down to sip cold water, I pulled out my phone and opened my inbox. There they were, about two hours of interviews with Marie and a historian named David Courtwright. My pulse quickened, and my eyes opened wide, a burst of energy replacing my afternoon slump. Throughout the rest of the training, I kept checking the clock eager to get back in my car and listen to Marie during my drive home.

I took the long way back to Tucson to give myself extra time and to guarantee that I'd pass a Dairy Queen; the pregnancy cravings

demanded ice cream. But the recordings were relatively old, from
the early 1980s, and I struggled to hear Marie over the car engine
and the whipping of the desert wind. I craned my head toward the
speaker, keeping my eyes on the highway ahead. It wasn't until I
was idling in the drive-through that I could truly appreciate the
warmth of her voice, gifted with an expansive emotional register
and frequent laughter.

Hearing Marie speak, I could now imagine her as an actual,
complete person instead of a mere abstraction. The photos I had
seen now came to life, imbued with her spirit. Her medical training
in the 1940s was not so different from my own. When asked what
she had learned about addiction in medical school, she responded,
"I don't think we were taught anything. There might have been a
few statements that addicts were terrible, or maybe one sneaked
into the hospital once." It wasn't until after her graduation, when
she was sent to work at the Lexington Narcotic Farm, that she first
knowingly saw someone with a substance use disorder. Decades
spanned between us; why had so little changed in our education?

Although the interviews resolved some of my questions, they
generated even more. What key details did not translate into the
interview itself, and why had they been excluded? When outlining
the shape of the negative space occupied by all the omitted details,
what could be seen?

Between 1980 and 1982, the man behind the microphone, David
Courtwright, interviewed Marie, Vince, and over sixty patients
who attended methadone clinics in New York City. Now he was
in his sixties, a retired professor of history at the University of
North Florida. In one black-and-white photo I found online, he
was tilting his head, wrinkling his forehead, and scratching his
short salt-and-pepper hair while wearing a dark suit jacket over a
white collared shirt—a mix of playful and academic. In another, he
was laughing, the coarse white stubble in his goatee and mustache
caught by the light. In another, he was serious, the orbits around
his eyes sunken and sullen.

I wanted to turn the microphone back on Courtwright, trans-
forming the one-sided interview into a dialogue that better illuminated the perspective through which Marie was examined. When he

asked Marie to explain why she used her maiden name to publish her pivotal work, *The Drug Addict as a Patient*, I felt offended on her behalf. It seemed obvious—Nyswander was the name she had built for herself, associated with decades of hard work, published papers, expertise. That, anyway, was the reason I had not changed my name, as was the simple fact that men were never asked to change theirs. Did she feel the same way?

Courtwright quickly responded to my initial email, saying he would be happy to talk, but, first, I should read a few more things. One, an eight-page article that he published about Marie in 1997. Two, a novel by her prior husband, Leonard Robinson, *The Man Who Loved Beauty*. Three, Leonard's notes about the book, held in his archives at the University of Montana. Courtwright also warned me, "Fasten your seatbelt before reading Robinson." It was good advice: his novel was a thinly veiled roman-à-clef depicting Marie as a naive, cockteasing goddess who is easily wooed by Vince's accolades and thus foolishly abandons the virtuous Robinson—that is, until Robinson wins her back through creepy stalking and the destruction of Vince's reputation. Then, Marie happily gives up her medical career to have babies. Although I am very thankful that real life ended differently, I doubt Robinson was. If that was the kind of pressure she faced from loved ones in her life, it is even more remarkable that she persevered.

The day of our virtual call, I put on a nice shirt, tucked my wild auburn curls behind my ears, and kicked my husband, Warren, out of our shared home office; nothing could interfere. When Courtwright's face—serious bordering on dour—appeared on my computer screen, I straightened my posture. But as we dove into the details of Marie's life and my plethora of questions, it felt more like we were in the middle of a casual conversation about a good friend. He smiled often, and my shoulders relaxed. He frequently asked my opinion, leaning in when the details got juicy. I felt like I could trust him.

"Welcome to the Marie Nyswander club," he beckoned. "This is really a small, elite club of people who just drive themselves crazy trying to figure her out." By the end of our conversation, he even promised to send me a box of all the files he collected when writing about Marie in the 1990s, including the notes he took during interviews with her family and ex-husband, the one and only Leonard Robinson. I couldn't believe my luck.

During the week that followed, I set up tracking notifications for his package on my phone. While waiting in line at the grocery store or even between patients in the emergency department, I obsessively checked the package's course as it traveled from Florida to Arizona. The day it was expected to arrive, I asked my husband to answer the door if someone knocked. Although he currently worked from home, he was usually too focused on his spreadsheets and computer models to pay attention to any distractions, his dark brown eyes peering through his glasses as his slim, tanned fingers clacked across his keyboard to adjust various formulas. Even if he weren't so engrossed in his analyses, the delivery driver's loud knock would be drowned out by his podcast soundtrack.

Later that afternoon, I was biking our two-year-old home from daycare when I saw the UPS truck pull away from the curb. I pushed my feet down harder, faster, against my pedals, the force of my velocity throwing my daughter back against her foam seat. The cardboard box was sandwiched between the iron storm door and the front wall of our house, and, although I immediately brought the box inside, I knew better than to open it around my inquisitive toddler. I wanted to keep the contents safe and pristine, to treat them with the respect they deserved. I knew much of the material within couldn't be reproduced, such as the handwritten interviews with people long gone. I hid the box in a high cabinet out of sight.

It wasn't until my daughter's nap a few days later that I finally opened the box, cutting away at the layers of packaging tape, pulling out piles of crumpled *Wall Street Journal* articles that had been used as padding, and unearthing two large manilla envelopes, each closed with a thick blue rubber band. One contained Courtwright's interview notes for his 1997 article about Marie for *Addiction*, and the other for his 1999 piece in *American National Biography*.

I wanted to look at every scribbled note in the margins, every clue, like the note Courtwright had written to himself: "My conviction grows that Marie needs more than 1,000 words. It turns out there may be a fourth husband, although I'm not sure about this."[16] At the time, he could only find evidence of three.

At the top of the stack were letters between Courtwright and the editors at *Addiction* regarding edits to his article. Most were simply pleasantries, but, in one, I found a suggestion that would come to haunt my entire journey with Marie.

The editor wrote, "I am still puzzled as to the precise role that Marie Nyswander played in the Dole/Nyswander achievements. When I've talked to Dole he has understandably always taken a deeply personal view on the brilliance, humanity, and historical significance of his wife's contributions and especially after her death no decent person would want to challenge this personal view. I have sometimes been left wondering whether Nyswander was in truth more important to Dole as a person than as a scientific collaborator, but I know that I could be radically and woefully wrong."

The audacity of such a claim! If anything, Marie was the one bringing more to the table in terms of addiction. She had decades of experience, several publications in reputable medical journals, a book that argued for the medical model of addiction, and, for years, had dreamed of prescribing opioids like methadone as treatment. Although they certainly benefited from Vince's prestige and research experience, his area of expertise was in metabolic diseases, a completely different field. Vince only became interested in addiction medicine in the early 1960s because a friend went on a sabbatical and asked him to take his place as chair of NYC's Committee on Narcotics. Realizing he knew nothing about addiction, he sought someone who did. That's when he found Marie.

Did the editor think that Marie had only married her way into success? Could he not believe that a woman was capable of such a monumental development, à la Rosalind Franklin? Although she was the scientist who discovered DNA's double helix, she did not receive any recognition during her lifetime; instead, the credit was awarded to her male partners. Or was he just reflecting how everybody else viewed her role? During my later interviews with people close to Marie, other men would echo the same suspicions. But I wouldn't let the issue drop; I owed at least that much to Marie, as well as to the women who are still to come. Until flawed histories are corrected to award credit where it is due, we cannot truly move forward.

To find the answers, I interviewed her close colleague and maid of honor, now ninety-six years old. I called the writer with whom she had dinner every weekend, and who was at the time in a realestate battle with Vince's third wife's son. Eventually, I was chatting with drug czars and DEA chiefs. At the height of this project, the characters began to invade my dreams. There was never a time when I wasn't thinking about Marie, about methadone, about the DEA. But, first, let's start at the beginning.

CHAPTER 2

The Beginning

1919–1933

In 1919, Marie was born in Reno, Nevada. Usually, I hated when biographies started at "the beginning," but in Marie's case, these were the kinds of details I craved. What about her early life preconditioned her for success and taught her to think outside the box? What could it teach me about becoming somebody whose work held the potential to change the world?

When Marie was two, her parents divorced, leaving her an only child. Her dad was a mathematician, and her mom a rancher's daughter-turned-graduate student. It wouldn't be until decades later, at her father's funeral in 1969, that she discovered she had a younger half-sister whose peals of laughter sounded just like her own.

Marie and her mom moved to the insular community of Alameda, a man-made island between San Francisco and Oakland where I would later work as an ED doc. They rented a room in a house owned by a young widow who had two children of her own and didn't mind babysitting Marie. That was a fortunate situation, as Marie's mom wasn't around much. After a full day of teaching at Alameda High School, she ran lab experiments late into the night while pursuing her PhD at Berkeley. Eventually, she would become a renowned researcher who helped found Berkeley's School of Public Health and frequently traveled abroad with the World Health Organization.

On the weekends, the voices of Marie's mom's radical friends filled the home, including Margaret Mead, Ruth Benedict, and Cora Du Bois—female anthropologists who shaped history at a time when few women were in academia. Margaret and Ruth also had a romantic relationship, something not socially acceptable in the 1920s. Marie told Nat Hentoff, a writer at *The New Yorker*, "They'd be sitting around the fireplace, talking about future research plans and trading ideas while I'd be under the piano, permitted to chip in my opinion whenever I wanted to. . . . Freedom and mobility, those were the characteristics of this family!" It all sounds so dreamy, the kind of environment I'm trying to curate for my own daughters.

Her mom was a bit wild, dragging Marie with her into the wilderness on camping trips. Once, they were camping in the mountains above Yosemite when a giant bear appeared. Her mom, "totally fearless," walked right up to the bear, "clapped her hands, told him to get away, and he did."[1]

On the surface, my childhood seemed quite different. I grew up in the small town of Huntsville, Alabama, my dad an analyst for the army and my mom staying home. We lived in a nondescript four-bedroom house on the white side of town. Sunday mornings were spent at the nearby Methodist church, followed by brunch at home. My parents were conservative and introverted; there were no queer academics hanging around our house, no camping trips with bears.

But, looking closer, there were certain similarities. I, too, was an only child, and even though our living room walls were lined with bookshelves, we frequently took family excursions to the library to accrue more. My dad filled his free time playing chess and discussing philosophy, while my mom sang and strummed her guitar. Our home bordered open land, and afternoons were spent exploring the forest by myself or with neighborhood friends, ducking under the trailing tendrils of poison ivy and dodging the sharp thorns of the overgrown blackberry bushes. Sometimes we took a break to ride our bikes along a tributary of the Tennessee River, stopping at the run-down gas station to buy orange sherbet push pops, our hair plastered with sweat across our sticky faces. Freedom and mobility: those were the characteristics of my family, too.

After Marie's mom finished her PhD, she accepted an offer at the University of Utah, and they moved to Salt Lake City. But when Marie was diagnosed with tuberculosis at age fourteen, she was sent, alone, to Southern California to live and heal at the Pottenger Sanatorium from 1933 to 1934. As it wasn't until 1949 that scientists discovered the real cure for tuberculosis—antibiotics—fresh air and relaxation were the only treatments available. Photos of the sanatorium show white wooden craftsman buildings topped by green gables, bordered on one side by the dry, scrub-green San Gabriel mountain range and by fruit trees and verdant lawns on the other. It was advertised as having the perfect climate in which to heal.

Compared to her childhood, I imagined that the isolated sanatorium must have felt extremely stodgy to teenage Marie, but she later described the experience as "marvelous" because she was introduced to so many new ideas. To fill the expansive hours, she listened to the radio and turned to books for entertainment.[2] For the first time, she heard classical music and jazz, two genres that would later become significant in her life. I like to imagine that the sanatorium's large compound had a sizable library, one so large that ladders were needed to reach the highest shelves, but maybe it was just a haphazard pile of books left by former patients. In any case, Marie was influenced by Thomas Mann's *The Magic Mountain*, which also took place in a tuberculosis sanatorium, and John Strachey's *The Coming Struggle for Power*, a socialist critique of capitalism that leaned heavy on Leninism.

One afternoon, Marie was lying in her cabin shaded by trees, listening to Louis Armstrong's deep voice and feeling the cool breeze through her screened windows, when she smelled something savory and heard a knock at her door—one of the staff members bringing her a choice cut of roast beef for dinner. Recalling Strachey, she wondered where poor people with tuberculosis recovered, as she doubted it was such an idyllic setting. Her doctor later confirmed her suspicions.[3]

Although Marie had been raised by a single mom in a board-inghouse, she did not consider herself poor—that probably didn't fit with the identity she had crafted for herself—and this unequal treatment of patients with tuberculosis became the first time she began to think about class, power, and social justice. In response, she decided to learn everything she could about Marx and Lenin.

Inside Strachey's book jacket, Marie noticed an address for a Los Angeles bookstore, and so, one night, she snuck out and somehow found her way there.[4] Did she hitchhike the twenty miles? Sneak a ride from another patient's family member? It was miraculous that she was able to locate the store at all, as it was unobtrusively located in an old building on a dark street. Maybe it was one of Los Angeles's clandestine communist bookstores.

Clandestine, because they were often targeted by police raids and FBI investigations.[5] Historian Joshua Clark Davis has described such bookstores as "one of the most important spaces for radicals in twentieth century America." At the time, communist theory often intermingled with labor organizing and civil rights, and so many politicians were quick to label anything that was progressive as communist. This was not a label to be taken lightly.[6] Communism was seen as such a threat to American democracy that Congress and state legislatures passed anti-syndicalism laws to expose communists and prevent labor organizing.[7]

When fourteen-year-old Marie stepped inside the bookshop, she found a group of men sitting around a table discussing a work of anthropology.[8] Instead of feeling out of place, she was awestruck. "I thought it was some kind of heaven," she recounted. "Those seedy-looking people were so involved in this heavy literature. I couldn't believe that these raggle-daggle men would be so intelligent. . . . I had all this adolescent wonder about what I had stumbled in on, and so from then on, I became very politically and socially aware."[9] She sounded like someone I would have wanted to be friends with: half nerd, half aspiring radical. Members of the Socialist Labor Party, the men happily shared political pamphlets with her.

Marie's subsequent radicalization was not simply a tangent to her medical career; rather, it was a precondition. Addiction medicine, both then and now, is a specialty focused on marginalized communities. During Marie's career, psychiatrists believed that addiction was indicative of a severe personality disorder, and most hospitals actively turned away patients if they were suspected addicts. The staff believed that people with addiction would trick them into giving them drugs, an error that might cost them their medical license. Additionally, most people thought that addiction fell under the purview of law enforcement, not healthcare. Some states even criminalized addiction itself—not just possession of drugs or paraphernalia—and would arrest someone if they had track marks. In California, the forerunner of naloxone was initially used as an agent of state control, with police forcing it upon suspected drug users. If the medication pushed them into withdrawal, it was used as court evidence of their addiction.[10]

When Marie was finally discharged from the sanatorium, she pursued her revolutionary ambitions by joining the rising farm worker movement. During their strikes, she passed out food, shuttled organizers in what she referred to as her mom's "capitalist car," and did whatever else an unskilled, enthusiastic teenager could. When she and her mom moved to New York a couple of years later, her activism continued. As she told Courtwright, "I joined something called the Young Communist League and the next thing I knew, we worked very hard to send a rifle to loyalist Spain."[11] Hearing this, I laughed. I imagined her mom didn't know that her teenage daughter was trying to smuggle arms out of the country, but, if she did, she probably would have been supportive, at least philosophically.

Pretty soon, the communists were calling Marie a "political anarchist," as she was interested in too many competing organizations— the Trotskyites, the Marxists, the Young Communists—and they asked her to leave. No longer welcome as a radical revolutionary, she decided college was the next best thing.

1937–1941

I was between patients at the methadone clinic when my inbox dinged with a new email. It was from an archivist at Sarah Lawrence

College, the prestigious women's college where Marie earned her undergraduate degree in 1941. I was pleasantly surprised—I had emailed her so long ago that I had since forgotten—and hopeful as to what slivers of information she might share. Because of the COVID-19 pandemic, their archives had been closed and their employees were working from home, but now that cases were falling in early 2021, the doors were not so firmly shut. Attached to the email were a few articles from their alumni magazine about Marie, as well as instructions for accessing old issues of their student newspaper, where Marie had served as a reporter. Excitedly, I scanned through the attachments and searched the newspaper archives for colorful anecdotes that could add depth to the bare scaffolding I had constructed thus far around her college years.

Old photographs revealed an idyllic campus: a hedge-lined road weaving between lush lawns and three-story brick Tudor buildings with steep roofs and multiple chimneys. According to Hentoff's biography, Marie felt free and supported to explore her interests in college, much as she had during childhood. Following the pedagogies of Oxford and Cambridge, the school had replaced large lecture halls with small seminars and one-on-one instruction. As she was their first premedical student, they even hired special faculty to teach her science prerequisites. Although she thought she had left her revolutionary days behind, they were only just beginning.

She came up frequently when I searched the archives for her name, partially because the paper read like a gossip column, and partially because she was fully engaged in her college experience. She was often listed alongside a friend of hers from Arizona, attending parties and football games with boys from the Ivies. The summer after her friend graduated, they took a road trip to her hometown in Tombstone, a dusty town ninety minutes from Tucson and best known for its daily reenactments of a nineteenth-century gunfight. When they were stuck on a dirt road in the middle of a summer monsoon, her friend said of the experience, "We were sure that we were going to die after being stuck in the desert for eleven hours with no food, no road and all rain. It was 150 miles to the nearest bit of habitation. It was luck and my strength that finally got us started again."[12]

Her friend had accepted a marriage proposal from a local boy, and they were on their way to meet him. However, when the rain dried up and they finally arrived, they discovered that not only had the fiancé lied about his impressive job, but he was unemployed. Right then and there, she broke up with him and kept driving west until she hit Hollywood, where she would sing in a night club and help a corporate tycoon write his autobiography.[13] Even Marie's friends were larger than life.

Another summer, Marie traipsed around Central America, getting stung by a stingray in Guatemala and bit by ants in Honduras. She was likely following in the footsteps of her adventurous mom; before Marie, she had trekked across the Sierras carrying no more than a rucksack full of potatoes for food and a homemade sleeping bag for shelter. When she was in her sixties, with failing vision, she happily slept on a rolled-up mat on the floor of a schoolroom in India.

Although Marie had retired from her stint as a communist, she was still politically active. She wrote several letters to the editor and an article condemning a senator's past involvement with the Ku Klux Klan. During her first Christmas vacation, she traveled to Vassar to represent Sarah Lawrence at the National American Student Union Convention and participated in a protest against Japan's invasion of China. Although she was one of five hundred other students, she was the one noticed by a national journalist. This was the first description of Marie that I found in the national press, back in 1937, back before she was *somebody*. She was barefoot in the snow, pulling off her silk stockings to throw into a campus bonfire. She and the other students chanted, "If you wear cotton, Japan gets nothin'."[14] Somehow, she stood out even then.

Recently, *The New York Times* ran an article about the moment when famous people were first mentioned in the news, often before they had done anything particularly noteworthy.[15] What about them drew attention? There was a photo of a young Patti Smith, months before the release of her debut album, standing in front of a barricade that reads, "Do not cross," a crowd of people behind her. Even in a crowd of people, "she [stood] out like the star she [would] become."[16]

As the authors wrote of this archival series, "You flip through these photographs and see authenticity and passion. They are more than portraits of people who are on the verge of becoming very successful and very famous. There's a pureness to these images. It feels like you are looking at people who are doing what they love, before the world was watching, and discovering who they are. This is a moment when things began to shift. They are in the process of becoming. . . There is a kind of magic that comes at the beginning of a journey." Obviously, the same could be said of young Marie. Did I have it, too?

It was easy to identify people as visionary and successful after they had achieved mainstream acceptance, but what about when they were still swimming upstream? When everyone else thought they were crazy? As someone who was at the beginning of my career, whose words and ideas were often met with skepticism that made me doubt myself, I was interested in what the process of becoming looked like. Not just in my career, but in life itself. Although I did not aspire to fame, I did want to step into my purpose, and it would be nice to have a little confirmation that I was on the right path.

In college, Marie initially set her sights on a musical career. She had been playing piano since she was three years old and was remarkably talented. In a 1939 issue of the campus paper, Marie confessed that her secret desire was to "play one measure better, faster, louder, and more perfectly than Mr. Haendl [sic]," the Baroque composer.[17] Unlike me, Marie seemed awfully cultured for a teenager, and it was by her own hand. It wasn't until her stay at the sanatorium that she first heard classical music, and now she was playing Baroque operas. Later, I would listen to interviews that suggested Marie carefully crafted her public persona, going as far as hanging particular art on her walls not because she liked it, but because it bolstered her image as a cultured New Yorker, a sharp contrast to her identity as a Californian raised by a rancher's daughter. And, based on these archives, her transformation had already begun. She even changed her name from Mary to the more exciting Marie, telling her mom, "There were too many Marys around the place," and that she "wanted a name with more character to it."[18]

Despite Marie's musical talent, she didn't think she was good enough to be a full-time composer, so she switched her ambitions toward medicine. Unlike a career in the arts, a career in medicine could be guaranteed. Work hard and perform the prescribed steps, and you would be a doctor. But in the arts, nothing was certain. Maybe you'd be good enough, maybe you'd catch a break, or maybe you wouldn't. Marie said, "It was clear that I certainly would have a ceiling [on my musical ability], whereas I couldn't see what ceiling would be applied to medicine, and so I think I took the avenue where I couldn't see the limitations."[19] It is amazing to me that in the 1930s, when only 5 percent of women were medical students, that she did not perceive a glass ceiling. Did she know any female doctors, making it easier to see herself as one? Or was it simply her mom's influence?

When Courtwright later asked if her mom's interest in public health affected her decision to become a physician, Marie answered, "Not to become a physician, but what I did with being a physician, I think. It seemed like being a Ph.D. was a very difficult and long and arduous thing and becoming an M.D. seemed much easier, so I just became an M.D. . . . but I think my interest in the public health aspect, the community aspect certainly, the great privilege of working in East Harlem, such an interest must have come from my mother."[20]

Marie told Hentoff, "I must have really known all the time that I was going to become a doctor. Medicine is such a compelling drive that I doubt if any doctor does have an actual second choice. I'm not sure why it's so compelling. Service. Prestige. Security. Independence. It must be a constellation of certain needs within yourself. I remember thinking that above all, I would be independent and could go wherever I wanted to."[21] As Marie had lived during the Depression and grown up with a single mom during a time when women were supposed to rely on their husbands, she understood the freedom that came with financial independence.

1941–1944

Marie applied to twenty medical schools and was accepted by all of them. Ultimately, she chose Cornell and began school in 1941, but she didn't bother to tell her mom until several months later. Her mom said this was evidence of how they "respected each other's independence," a unique aspect of their relationship that came up in my research over and over again.[22] During this time, her mother remarried and moved back to California to help found Berkeley's College of Public Health, now one of the most distinguished programs in the world.

I wanted to know more about Marie's medical school experience, but the records were scarce. I could only ascertain five things: 1) she graduated in an accelerated time frame, in three years instead of four, because of World War II; 2) many of her classmates joined the military upon graduation out of a sense of patriotism, and she, too, wanted to serve her country; 3) she was briefly married to one of her anatomy and physiology instructors, Charles Berry; 4) she claimed that sexism did not exist; and 5) she planned to become an orthopedic surgeon.

The marriage was not something Marie often talked about, not even to her closest friends. When I brought it up to Dr. Joyce Lowinson, a physician who worked closely with Marie at Rockefeller and served as her bridesmaid when she married Vince, she responded, "She had said Leonard [Robinson] wasn't the first but never discussed Charles Berry, and I didn't prod." When Courtwright referred to Leonard as her first husband, Marie didn't correct him.

It wasn't until a decade later, after Marie's death, when Courtwright learned of this secretive affair. He was completing research for her biography, and Vince recommended that he speak with Marie's mom. Although she was ninety-eight years old, Vince said "she still had most of her marbles" and would have a lot of good personal information to share. So, Courtwright called her up for an interview, unprepared for the surprises to come.

First of all, her mom kept referring to her as Mary, not Marie. That's when Courtwright learned that Marie had changed her name in college. Then her mom said that Marie's first husband was a "nice chap" named Charles Berry, not Leonard. Marie was just twenty-four when they wed, and the union only lasted two years. Marie's mom wasn't sure why they divorced; Marie never told her. A trained historian, Courtwright searched for additional proof of this clandestine marriage and found it in Cornell's records. According to some facts Courtwright scribbled on a piece of notebook paper, Cornell listed Marie's last name as Nyswander from 1942 to 1943, but as Berry from 1943 to 1944.

Later, I would learn that Charles Berry wasn't even her first husband. When she was just sixteen, she married a premedical student in Utah named Gordon Woodrow Raleigh, but the marriage didn't last long. According to newspaper announcements, Gordon remarried within the next year. If Marie's mom knew anything about this marriage, she certainly didn't let on. It was only through transcripts of interviews that I found hints of its existence, and it was my genealogy-buff uncle who ultimately helped me find the marriage announcements on Ancestry.com.

I could think of many reasons why Marie would carefully hide these marriages from the world at large. At the time, divorce was more stigmatized and less common. Perhaps she felt like each marriage also cheapened the dedication she felt to her current husband. Moreover, on a professional level, Marie began her career as a marital psychiatrist. How could she be seen as an expert if she herself had several "failed" marriages? It would jeopardize her credibility. And as one of the few women in medicine, I'm sure she had even less wiggle room in that regard.

But why did she hide these relationships from her friends and family? I, too, had been married more than once. When I was twenty, I eloped with an engineering student from Kenya. Although I felt a little silly when I told people about this, as it now seemed a rash, youthful decision, I did not regret it. He was the one who first convinced me I could become a doctor, the one who pushed me to aspire for more. But, unlike Marie, I had a tendency to keep things a little "too real," the opposite of her careful construction of an outward-facing identity.

I also could not relate to her assertions that sexism was non-existent at Cornell. About ten minutes into their 1981 interview,

Courtwright asked her, "Were you self-conscious about being a female medical student at Cornell?" I imagined them sitting in her Rockefeller office, jazz records and medical tomes lining her bookshelves, and a classical piano score sitting on her desk alongside the latest issue of the *New England Journal of Medicine*.[23] Listening to the tapes, I could hear a frequent high-pitched beeping in the background, like something out of a sci-fi movie from the seventies. Marie quickly responded to Courtwright's question, not needing even a second to think, "Mm, mm, no, I don't think anybody was." Did she meet his gaze when she said this? Did she really believe it, or was it just that she wanted to?

I imagine him sitting in a chair across from her, legs crossed, leaning back. At this point, he had conducted almost a hundred such interviews for his book of oral histories related to the heroin epidemic of the 1970s, and he was familiar with the process of pulling uncomfortable information from strangers. He pressed further: "How was the composition of your class? Were you the only woman? One of a few women?"

"I think we had two or three, three I think." She answered. I could not even imagine this; in my class of almost two hundred, we had been nearly fifty-fifty. How did she navigate being one of the only women in her class? If it were me, I probably would have downplayed my femininity, trying to blend in. To be feminine was to be associated with a litany of unfavorable characteristics, especially in medicine: unintelligent, emotional, submissive, weak, uncommitted, indecisive. As the medical director of several fire departments, I wore a navy polo shirt and loose slacks when I met with the crews. I didn't wear any makeup, and I pulled my hair into a bun. Nationwide, 96 percent of firefighters were male, and I didn't want to stand out any more than I already did. I felt grateful that I was thin and not particularly curvy.

But, for all I have read about Marie, I doubt that downplaying her femininity was her method. I imagine her instead choosing to stand out, wearing bracelets that slid down her slim wrists when she raised her hand to speak, using her wit and infectious smile to charm her classmates and professors alike. She was confident and strategic enough to use her sexuality to her advantage. According to Charles Winick, a sociologist with whom she worked, she had a "Bette Davis Complex and wasn't afraid to flaunt it"—Bette Davis, the critically acclaimed actress who alternated between charming and brash, cigarette in hand.[24] And if the depictions in Leonard Robinson's novel were accurate, Marie, too, was a bit of a seductress.

But, certainly, Marie must have faced some level of sexism. I know I had: when I witnessed a supervising attending physician griping, "This is why we shouldn't have female residents," in response to a coresident deciding to take four months of maternity leave, even though she still had to make up those months and prolong her graduation date. When, during an EMS fellowship interview, the program director warned me that the fire departments wouldn't listen to me because I was a woman; they had upper-body strength requirements, after all. When I almost didn't graduate on time from residency because my attendings gave me low scores on their assessment of my leadership abilities—an occurrence that is common for female residents.[25] When I decided to delay parenthood until after my medical training, a decision shared by most of the female physicians I knew but none of the men. When I had to pump in the emergency department's sexual assault exam room because there was nowhere else available for me, storing the milk for my daughter next to rapists' sperm. When a physician I supervised left a shift early and provided substandard care to several patients, and then said I was the one with the problem because I tried to hold him accountable. But even worse were the ways in which sexism affected our patients, such as the time when a patient's blood pressure dropped dangerously low because she was hemorrhaging into her belly while the physician caring for her discounted her pain as hysteria, missing the ruptured ectopic pregnancy that threatened to kill her. All of this in the twenty-first century.

A growing body of research suggests that I am not alone: sexism in medicine is a systemic problem. Women medical students are more likely than men to experience microaggressions.[26] When applying to the male-dominated field of orthopedic surgery, women applicants are more likely to be asked about family planning, a question topic that the American College of Graduate Medical Education clearly classifies as illegal.[27] In formal evaluations of emergency medicine residents, men receive higher scores on their mandatory milestones while women receive more negative feedback around their receptivity to guidance,[28] yet, at the same time, are criticized for their lack of assertiveness.[29] Even in the female-dominated field of obstetrics and gynecology, women residents receive lower ratings, less positive feedback, and more negative feedback from nurses.[30] After training ends, women physicians make $20,000 less than their male equivalents, even when adjusted for hours worked.[31] Despite the lower evaluations and lower pay, studies also suggest that women physicians are just as good at their jobs as men, if not better, theorizing that sexism, not an actual difference in quality, is the root of the inequalities.[32] So don't expect me to believe that sexism didn't exist in Marie's 1940s.

Was Marie just being precise with her words? Perhaps she meant that it wasn't medical school where she faced discrimination, but, later, when she tried to practice clinically. After all, the sexism I faced in medicine only seemed to worsen as my career ascended. I hardly faced any issues in medical school and, because of this, subtly felt that sexism was something we had long overcome in medicine. In residency, things got a little worse. Then when I was a medical director, they got a lot worse. The more power I obtained, the more upset people became.

Yet Marie was not the only one who denied the existence of sexism in medicine. A 1947 issue of Sarah Lawrence's alumni newspaper profiled a premedical student who graduated four years after Marie. Herself a college senior heading to medical school in a few months, she said, "This group is the largest class of women medical students the College has ever had, and there isn't any chance of prejudice against us." Because of Marie's example, it was no longer abnormal to be a premedical student at Sarah Lawrence. She had paved the way. The student continued, "All it takes to get through medical school is stick-to-itiveness, a tough fanny for sitting at lectures, and strong legs for getting from class to class."[33]

When I asked Dr. Joyce Lowinson about Marie's assertions about equality, she believed that Marie had meant what she said. Furthermore, she felt the same way: "I knew there was sexism, but I didn't experience it. I didn't think about it."

Because there were so few women in medicine, perhaps their presence was more tolerated. They were a curiosity of sorts. Additionally, they probably weren't trying to change the system to make it more equitable; they were too busy just trying to make it through. Or maybe denial was the only way they found the strength to keep going.

Could Marie's sexism denial also be part of the image she was trying to portray to the world? I imagine it was an unpopular move in medicine, as well as in society at large, to claim that sexism existed. Americans like to think that we have moved beyond sexism, racism, ableism, antisemitism—it feels good to believe this myth, especially if you have benefited from it. If she wanted the public, especially those in power, to like her, it would be safest to collude with hegemony and play to the politics of assimilation. Not only that, but she would be praised for doing so. The patriarchy can only be upheld if it has female supporters.

But perhaps Marie wouldn't have been able to accomplish all that she did without some level of pandering. Although she had a lot of privileges that helped open doors—whiteness, education, connections to powerful people and institutions—she was still trying to wield power within spaces that were carefully gatekept. If she wanted to be accepted within these structures that were designed to exclude her, she had to "pass" enough to gain, and then keep, her entry. Although she ultimately disrupted the system from the inside, there was still a ceiling to her level of subversion.

Back in Marie's Rockefeller office, Courtwright continued to push the issue, "You encountered no form of discrimination or ...?"

"No," Marie answered with warmth in her voice, the diction of the single word prolonged enough for her tone to drop. It sounded as if this were the first time she had been asked this particular question, and she was trying her best to answer earnestly. "No, I don't think so, well, one doctor, but he might just have not liked me or something, but otherwise no, I wouldn't say so." She paused. "I don't think any woman doctor would, uh, encounter. . . . I suppose if you applied for a job in which there was no ladies' room or no quarters to sleep in"—and, at this point, a deep laugh bubbled into her answer: "If it was on a destroyer you might have trouble," as if this were perfectly acceptable. If a hospital today refused to hire a woman because they didn't have a women's bathroom, a lawsuit would be just around the corner. But Marie couldn't even conceptualize a world in which a hospital or navy ship might accommodate women. I also don't know why she was laughing, as it didn't seem particularly funny. Was it just a tactic to cover up the pain? After all, this was exactly what happened to her.

CHAPTER 3

Bupísta

2017

The Highland Emergency Department was a maze of rooms and hallways, each haphazardly tacked on to the original Art Deco building during a series of add-on construction projects. Some patients lay in stretchers in the hallways, others in large rooms cordoned off by curtains, and a lucky few had their own rooms. Today, I was working a shift on the half of the department dedicated to the patients who triage deemed less sick, which often included patients with psychiatric illness. Outside the large room that had become the de facto psychiatric unit, the other doctors and I shared a small counter complete with six computers and a few less stools. Most of the time, it was fairly quiet, but sometimes our conversations were interrupted by shouting, police running down the hall to restrain someone, or patients wandering over to ask for somewhere more peaceful to rest. The emergency department was a harsh place.

Now that I was finished with residency and fellowship, Highland was my favorite place to work. As a county hospital, Highland embraced anyone and everyone who sought her care, offering a blend of dignified social justice and a whole lot of grit. The old-timers, docs and nurses who had worked there for years or even decades, were the stuff of legends. TV shows and full-length documentaries had been made about that ED, yet the truly wild stories remained unfilmed: wrestling matches at motorcycle gang headquarters, stolen propofol to sedate friends with broken bones from said matches, and bodies shoved down trash chutes. Sometimes the protagonists were the patients, sometimes the staff. Their emergency department also hosted a prestigious residency program, attracting some of the best medical students from around the country. As I was an attending physician, it was my job to supervise them.

I was sitting on a swivel stool with a cracking black cushion, clicking through a patient's chart, when one of the residents walked out of a side room and joined me. "I saw a patient in opioid withdrawal," he began, "with the classic symptoms of body aches, vomiting, diarrhea, diaphoresis, dilated pupils, piloerection, and agitation."

His words were interrupted by the sound of a man yelling obscenities punctuated by violent retching.

"Oh, that's him." The resident nodded. A nurse walked swiftly toward the patient's room, a crinkly blue emesis bag in hand.

"Anyway, his last use of heroin was yesterday, and he wants to stop using. I'd like to give eight milligrams of buprenorphine, reassess in thirty minutes, and perhaps give another twenty-four milligrams."

I heard the nurse call out to us: "Please, for the love of God, give him something. This guy is a mess." And then, to the patient: "Man, why did you throw up all over the floor? Couldn't you have tried to at least make it to the trash?" To be fair, he was sharing the room with about three other patients.

Not only had I never ordered buprenorphine, but I had only just heard of it a few months ago during a toxicology lecture.[1] I asked the resident beside me, "What is the typical dose of that medication? And what is the criteria for giving it?"

Josh Luftig, one of the physician assistants, was standing across from us at the raised counter, furiously typing into the computer. When he heard my question, he looked up from his screen, and the keys stopped clacking. He pushed back his short brown hair and asked, "Oh, you haven't given bupe yet?" Excitement glimmered across his face.

"No, I haven't."

He gave a short laugh, almost a chortle, and fanned his palms outward. "Prepare to be amaaaazed."

Josh had worked at Highland for years and seemed to know everything. He was the right-hand man of Dr. Andrew Herring, a surfer-turned-ED doc who was triple-boarded in emergency medicine, ultrasound, and, more recently, addiction medicine. Together, he and Josh had convinced everyone at Highland that addiction treatment was both a core component of emergency medicine and simple to provide. Among the throngs of patients easily treated and streeted in our fast track for runny noses, work notes, and infected hangnails, patients in opioid withdrawal were getting buprenorphine and sent out the door. It was revolutionary.

Josh confirmed that the resident's plan was a good one, and the order was placed. Thirty minutes later, I walked over to see how the patient was doing. At first, I thought I was in the wrong room. Instead of a surly man throwing up on the floor, there was a man cheerfully talking on the phone. Instead of wearing a crumpled hospital gown, he was dressed in a button-down shirt and navy slacks. He looked up at me as he spoke into the phone held in front of his mouth. "Hold on, one of the docs just walked in." He smiled and rested the phone in his lap.

"How are you feeling?" I asked.

"Normal!" he exclaimed, life bursting from his brown eyes.

"Really?" I rested my weight on my right foot, left hand on my hip.

"Yeah, and it feels great! I haven't felt like this in forever." He paused. "You know, using lately hasn't been fun anymore—I just use so I don't get sick. It's not like I get high anymore."

Although things normally hummed along at a brisk pace in the emergency department, never before had I seen a single treatment cause such a swift and total metamorphosis. Even if my actions had eventually prevented someone from dying, they were usually still too sick by the time they left the ED to realize what our team had done: the quick puncture of skin as IVs slid into their flattened veins, the rapid infusion of fluids and antibiotics into their body, the medications that constricted their vessels just enough to allow blood to reach their brain, heart, and kidneys. Collectively, all of these actions slowly beat back death, allowing the person in front of us more days in this shimmering, wild life—but all that took time.

Marie had experienced similar shock when watching methadone transform her patients. Usually, recovery was a series of fits and starts, a process marked by relapse. I'm sure the man in front of me also knew this, had lived this. And now, to have a medication that so smoothed the way—it must have felt miraculous.

His eyes looked directly into mine. "Thank you so much."

I laughed awkwardly and looked down. I was not usually the recipient of such sincere gratitude from patients; that just wasn't how the ED worked.

He wrapped his index finger and thumb around the top button of his shirt and splayed his other fingers across his chest. "Do you think you guys can hurry up and discharge me? I'd like to get going."

My eyes opened wider. Not only had buprenorphine helped this man, but it had helped our department. Whereas an hour ago, he was so sick that his nurse could barely care for her other patients, now he was antsy to leave, leaving an open bed in his wake. In ED terms, this was a remarkably quick dispo, something we strived for. There were always more patients who needed to be seen, and, at Highland, the wait could be hours.

When I returned to my computer station, Josh asked me, "Well, what do you think?"

"That was incredible!" I exclaimed.

He laughed. "Welcome to the club."

"How does it work?" I asked.

"It's a partial opioid agonist," he answered, "with a higher affinity for the mu-opioid receptor than other full-agonists."

If you remember the analogy of the ball and cup from earlier, where bupe is a ball floating toward the cup of the opioid receptor, now add a super strong magnetic charge to them both. This illustrates bupe's high affinity.

"Because of this," he continued, "patients need to be in opioid withdrawal when they get their first dose of bupe."

When our patient arrived in withdrawal, all of his receptors were empty. As the strip of bupe dissolved under his tongue, molecules absorbed across the pearly pink mucosa and into his bloodstream, hurtling toward the brain's opioid receptors. Once there, the machinery of his body breathed a collective sigh of relief.

Josh continued, "If they aren't in withdrawal first, bupe can precipitate it." He raised both eyebrows. "Which sucks."

Later, I would see a woman who had thrown herself into this suboptimal state after taking a strip of bupe from the street without any understanding of how it worked. Because it had just been a few hours since her last shot of heroin, her opioid receptors were still occupied. When bupe arrived, its higher affinity pushed heroin out of the way. But, because bupe was only a partial agonist, its downstream effects were not as strong as heroin's, and her body was catapulted into withdrawal as if she were a racecar driver slamming on the breaks. Her withdrawal was worse than I had ever seen before or since, her yells of agony audible from rooms away. She would probably never try buprenorphine again.

"To prevent this," Josh added, "it has to be at least twelve hours since their last use, and you need to actually see signs of withdrawal." In the years that followed, doctors would come up with other ways to start buprenorphine that did not require patients to suffer any withdrawal beforehand, but we didn't know that then.

I nodded. Relative to all the other complicated procedures we learned to perform in emergency medicine—like using a giant steel retractor to spread open someone's ribs before squeezing a gloved hand in the narrow space between the spine and heart to grasp the thick, flat tubing of a sheared aorta—this was easy. And, in terms of starting MOUD, I came to believe that not only was the emergency department a suitable alternative to a methadone clinic, but superior. Most methadone clinics had limited hours and only accepted certain insurance plans, and some were so backed up that it took weeks to secure an available appointment. If it was 5 p.m. on a Friday when somebody decided to quit, good luck. Because the stages of change were shaped like a circle, not a straight line, we might only have a narrow window in which to help someone who was ready to quit. If we missed our opportunity, fentanyl would be there, waiting. In contrast, the ED was open twenty-four hours a day, seven days a week, and we treated anyone who crossed our threshold, regardless of their ability to pay. When someone was ready, we were, too. Unfortunately, most docs did not agree, with only a smattering of emergency departments across the country offering this life-saving treatment.

Over the months that followed, I gave bupe to more and more patients, each administration further converting me into a bona fide *Bupísta*. Buprenorphine completely transformed the dynamic of my interaction with patients who used drugs. Finally, I had something to offer. Finally, we were on the same page. Instead of patients storming out the door too soon, patients hugged me with tears of joy running down their cheeks. If that sounds dramatic, it's because it is.

Critics might argue that my patients were grateful simply because I had provided them with the drug they were craving. But, just as Marie saw that methadone was not the same as heroin, I saw that neither was bupe. Instead of constantly focusing on the next fix, people taking MOUD now had the space to focus on living: going to school, spending time with family, working, and even thriving. Research showed that patients on these medications were more than twice as likely to remain in recovery, and, thus, alive.

Furthermore, it was possible that the positive experience of receiving MOUD might encourage ambivalent patients to seek treatment down the road. In an interview with *The New York Times*, Andrew Herring said of bupe and recovery, "You've given them a chance to test-drive it," he said. "They'll still remember in a month, in a year."[2] Buprenorphine was magic. Starstruck by bupe's potential, I saw treatment as the ultimate goal. Only later would I realize that harm reduction, both as a practice and a philosophy, might be even more powerful.

Pizza and beer in hand, I climbed the rickety wooden stairs to find a quieter location for our book club. The first to arrive, I set my greasy paper plate on a picnic table in the corner. The air smelled like cheese, tomato sauce, and freshly baked bread. I reached to turn down the sound on the television tacked to a nearby wall, as I didn't want our group to shout as we discussed tonight's book, Sam Quinones's *Dreamland*, a fast-paced narrative about our country's most recent opioid epidemic.

Increasingly interested in addiction medicine, I wanted to find more ways to incorporate it into my career. Sure, I was now giving buprenorphine during my shifts, but at the end of the day, I was still a burned-out emergency medicine doc going from shift to shift. Medicine as practiced in the real world felt much different than the version I had learned during training. For one, most emergency medicine doctors were hired by giant medical conglomerates owned by private equity, not nonprofit hospitals or independent physician groups, and we were encouraged to maximize the profits accrued from each patient encounter. At mandatory meetings, we learned tips and tricks to claim higher reimbursement rates, such as ordering a medication as an injection instead of a pill because it paid more. This was not why I had become a physician. I had wanted to make a difference in the world, à la Dr. Paul Farmer, the global health physician who believed that social justice was as central to healthcare as X-rays and medications.

Instead, I left most shifts feeling like I hadn't accomplished anything. Ordering a CT scan, telling a patient they weren't dying but I didn't know what exactly was causing their abdominal pain, and sending them out the door wasn't very satisfying. And when homeless patients checked into the ED because it was raining, there was no way I could provide what they really needed: a safe home, a living wage. But such was the practice of emergency medicine.

All of this was exacerbated by the fact that I didn't have one full-time job, instead patching together shifts at a handful of emergency departments across the Bay. Because I didn't spend much time at any one hospital, none felt like home. I constantly felt like a guest in someone else's house, nobody noticing if I wasn't there. It also meant that my shifts jumped erratically from days to nights to swings. During 4 a.m. commutes home, I sometimes fell asleep in the stop-and-go traffic of San Francisco rush hour.

Even though I had promised Warren that I would have more time for him once residency was over, it seemed like I was always too tired. I'm sure he missed the lively woman he had fallen in love with years ago, the one who knew how to squeeze adventures into life's every nook and cranny. But he never said anything; he was too kind. Our exploits withered from weeklong road trips to a dinner here, a dinner there. How many more years could our relationship sustain such neglect before we drifted out of love?

I had reached a kind of plateau that I didn't know how to escape. For years, I had been dutifully following the steps that, when performed well, guaranteed success: premed courses, MCAT, volunteer work, medical school, Step 1, Step 2, residency, chief year, fellowship. And now, for the first time in my life, there was no longer a clearly prescribed path to follow. It felt like I was floundering.

Hearing creaks on the staircase, I looked up just as Dr. Andrew Herring, our invited guest speaker, waved hello. I was surprised he agreed to join us, as my meager book club felt like quite a divergence from his usual speaking engagements at national conferences and in front of the National Institute on Drug Abuse.

He sat across from me and asked, "Hey, did I get here early?"

I smiled with false assurance. "Oh, no, it's the right time, but sometimes people show up a little late." I took a long drink from my beer, hoping the alcohol would ease my anxiety. I felt sheepish for not even buying his meal—he was probably used to paid flights and hotels.

Andrew smiled and used his long fingers to sweep hair out of his eyes. "Okay, great."

He was somewhat of a celebrity in our emergency department, and perhaps the world at large. It was rumored that, when he was surfing, he once pulled a drowning man out of the ocean and performed CPR right there on the beach. A modern-day hero. During ED shifts, Andrew would casually mention how the NIH had flown him across the country to teach experts about the opioid epidemic. He was a visionary. When he spoke, residents and nurses listened, no questions asked. In contrast, when I made similar claims, nurses often found another doctor for a second opinion, and residents asked me to cite my sources. In the silence between us, I worried what Andrew would think of me if nobody showed up. If the book club was a bust, would he ever take another chance on me? Secretly, I hoped that he might take me under his wing.

As I saw my friend's shaggy hair appear over the stairwell, I smiled and gesticulated wildly for her to join us. I had never been so happy to see her. Although more people arrived, most of the conversation bounced between Andrew and a graduate student who volunteered with the city's largest naloxone distribution program. As usual, Andrew focused on buprenorphine's potential, seeing it as the antidote to the spiraling epidemic described in *Dreamland*. Recently, he had even started to work for a local startup that offered buprenorphine via telemedicine, and he spoke excitedly about its potential to reach more people.

Like most states, large swaths of rural California lacked providers with a DEA-x license, the credential required until 2023 to prescribe buprenorphine.[3] Although it was easy for doctors to prescribe oxycodone, the medication that had become notorious for creating an entire new generation of people with addiction, it was so much harder to prescribe its treatment. Nurse practitioners had to take a twenty-four-hour course before they could apply for their DEA-x, and physicians eight. Many of my colleagues were scared off by such requirements, assuming that only a dangerous medication would need so much training. Others just didn't have the time to spend. Some saw telemedicine as a quick fix to this treatment desert, as it allowed patients to see a prescriber anywhere, anytime, no need to drive six hours to reach the nearest provider with a DEA-x.

Unfortunately, pivoting to telemedicine was not so easy. In 2008, the Ryan Haight Act mandated that a doctor had to see a patient in person before they could prescribe buprenorphine; telemedicine did not count. Ironically enough, this act was designed to combat the rogue online pharmacies that sold controlled substances like oxycodone and hydrocodone, the very drugs whose addiction buprenorphine could help treat.

But, as a physician, I wasn't sure why regulators thought we needed to physically examine a patient in order to diagnose them with opioid use disorder. Over a video visit, I could easily see the exam findings that I cared about, like the restless legs, dilated pupils, goosebumps, sweating, and yawning of withdrawal, or the sedation, pinpoint pupils, and slow respirations of intoxication.

Although we discussed some of the ways in which regulation hindered patients' access to treatment, I doubt we talked much about the regulatory risks of providing telemedicine. Based on other conversations with Andrew, I imagine he glazed over any potential hazards, not wanting to scare off future converts. For him, this technique worked. When I later tried it, people were rightfully suspicious. They asked for proof, wanting me to list specific regulations that might affect them. When I turned to Andrew, asking where I might find such answers, he simply waved his hand. Perhaps he saw me as just another doctor whose unorthodox methods caused them to make excuses.

Equally absent from the conversation was any mention of buprenorphine's forerunner, methadone. Because of its pharmacology, methadone is more likely than buprenorphine to interact negatively with other medications. And, because methadone is a full agonist, it is possible to overdose on it; thus, it is more heavily regulated. Although methadone can also be started in an emergency department, it cannot be prescribed from one. Regulations forbid pharmacies from dispensing methadone to treat addiction (although they can dispense it for "pain"), so patients with opioid use disorder have to go to a certified methadone clinic every day to receive their daily dose. In contrast, buprenorphine can be picked up at any pharmacy, anywhere. Because of this, Andrew did not see a future for methadone. Similarly, Josh later wrote me, "In the ED, it's all bupe, all the time."

Later, I would learn that there were also racial overtones to medicine's preference for buprenorphine. Although buprenorphine was developed as a pain medication in 1966, its potential in treating addiction wasn't fully recognized until the 1990s, a time when the face of opioid addiction had become overwhelmingly white.[4] Prescription drug use, primarily oxycontin, was soaring, especially in the suburbs and rural America. But instead of treating these users as immoral or criminal, they were seen as victims. As such, they deserved a more convenient treatment, one they could get from their family doctor's office. Methadone was positioned as the treatment for urban, Black and Brown users, and buprenorphine for whites. Suboxone's advertising amplified this divergence, highlighting the stories of middle-class white people whose lives had been ruined by something as wholesome as a football injury.

As the hour drew to a close, Andrew drank the last sips of his beer and told us how the startup he worked for was looking for more docs to join their team. The blur caused by my drink quickly faded, an alertness now thrumming. I'd love to be a telemedicine addiction doc. I wrote down the contact info he shared, and, with that, he stood up, smiled, and jaunted toward the exit. My body sank with relief into the bench, glad the performance was over. I hated how self-conscious I felt around him, how I held him up on a pedestal, how I longed for him to take an interest in my career. Looking back now, the entire scene makes me wince—I was so bumbly, so un- polished, so eager! Can't I just forget this awkward book club ever happened? As this younger version of myself is such a contrast to my current professional identity—one in which I'm running our hospital's addiction service, working closely with our county and state health departments, speaking at national presentations, men- toring fellows, writing research papers—it feels like a dream where your spirit separates from your body and watches all the strange things that some other character does. But it wasn't somebody else; it was me: vulnerable, embarrassed, and a little lost. Maybe that is just how the process of becoming looks.

As my friend and I bused our table, she told me, "One of my friends started a similar telemedicine company and they are looking for a doc to be their chief medical officer."

My lips curved with curiosity. "Oh, yeah?" I asked. "Could you introduce us?" Being a CMO with a startup offered everything I had been looking for: Addiction medicine. Leadership. Purpose. Learning something new. Providing a life-saving treatment. Breaking down barriers. And, when in the Bay . . . joining a startup seemed like the thing to do.

Wanting to make a good impression, I showed up early for my interview with the two CEOs. Their California office was just a few blocks from our townhouse, tucked inside a yellow stucco loft building with a bizarrely columned front archway that looked like it was straight out of the late eighties, complete with a bright red door and yellow columns topped with black pyramids. It was reminiscent of Willy Wonka's Chocolate Factory. But when my phone rang, I realized that there had been no need to drive over. The interview would not be in person, but via video chat. Of course, how foolish of me. They were a tech company, after all, and one of their CEOs worked from their Michigan office.

I answered, already a little flustered by my misunderstanding. Surely they saw the car headrest behind me, but did they see the beads of sweat on my upper lip? The faces of the two CEOs flashed on-screen, both young women also in their thirties. One was gregarious and friendly, the other a little more reserved, a characteristic I always found intimidating. One said something along the lines of "I'm not sure how much you've heard about us, but we can start with a brief introduction." When one paused, the other seamlessly took over. This pitch was not their first.

"We are both in recovery ourselves, and, knowing how difficult treatment can be, we want to make the experience as pleasant as possible for our patients."

"I had been to so many AA meetings where lecherous old men tried to take advantage of young women and the vulnerability of nascent sobriety, and to clinics that felt more like jails than healing environments."

"We want to create a new experience of addiction treatment, one that feels like you are stepping into a spa or yoga studio. One that is easy for the client and meets their unique needs. It is the antithesis of a methadone clinic."

"And we want to make it affordable. We are applying for a grant that will let us treat most patients for free, and the rest on a sliding scale."

"We are a certified B corp, which means we follow certain ethical business practices, and we have received series A funding."

I nodded, as if I knew what that meant, but I had no idea. This was my first interlude with a startup and its associated business jargon.

"Only 1 percent of companies who have received series A funding are run by women."

I yearned to be a part of their team, to join a female-dominated C-suite.

"We currently just have a clinic in Michigan, but as we expand to California, we want a physician to play more of a leadership role, someone who has the same values. Someone who wants to make treatment easier and more accessible."

I nodded. Although I had very little experience with buprenorphine at this point, it seemed like something I could figure out relatively quickly. If Highland's ED fast track gave it out, surely it couldn't be that difficult.

Additionally, I was already talking with Josh and Andrew about converting their method into a formulaic algorithm similar to the protocols that paramedics and EMTs used daily. Although many docs thought their medical decision-making was too complex to be captured by a simplistic flow chart, I found that if I asked enough questions, I could usually translate their thought process into a simple decision tree. Bupe protocol in hand, doctors around the country would have the benefit of Josh and Andrew's expertise, and many more patients could be reached. It would be easy for me to modify this protocol for a telemedicine setting.

I jumped in: "All of this sounds like a wonderful opportunity and like a good fit. How are you navigating the regulations posed by the Ryan Haight Act? The one that mandates a first visit in person?"

"Good question. We will open a brick-and-mortar clinic where patients can come for their first visit. Initially, it will probably be just one day a week, but as we expand, so will the days. Subsequent visits can be done via telemedicine. We are also going to hire nurse practitioners to be the primary clinical providers. Your role would be more on big picture stuff, as well as overseeing the nurse practitioners." I squirmed with the excitement of possibility.

In a few weeks, the CEOs offered me the position. It didn't pay particularly well, my hourly rate less than one-third of what I earned in the ED, but I didn't mind. The job offered something more than money—satisfaction. Alongside a team of pioneering young women, I was given the opportunity to change a broken system. And, for the first time, I felt that my bosses recognized my potential. Reflected in their eyes, I reveled in my new identity as the ideas person.

One day a week, we rented a small, shabby office on the eastern side of the Berkeley Hills that belonged to a child psychologist. We were not allowed to change the decor, so the only art hanging on the wall was a framed illustration of a creepy, lonely child. The office shared its bathroom with a small insurance company and a business that provided some kind of shipping service, so after our patients left their urine sample on the counter by the sink, we quickly ran in to dip the bendy drug-testing strip into their pee before anybody else walked in. We didn't want to be kicked out as soon as we arrived.

As our company was in its infancy, we knew it would take time (and money) to grow a client base that justified a real clinic building. Besides, our patients only had to set foot in here once before their care was moved online. Despite the odd setting, there was nowhere else I wanted to be. Every time I pulled into the parking lot, excitement buoyed me into the building. A social worker, nurse practitioner, and I were the only staff, and everything we did felt important. Together, we were building something special. I imagined this was how Marie felt when working alongside Dr. Beatrice Berle, a family medicine physician who invited Marie to join her East Harlem clinic in 1958.

In contrast to the punitive vibe of many addiction clinics, we wanted our patients to feel valued. As people who use drugs face stigma in almost every aspect of their lives, we aspired to provide a kind of sanctuary. We also tried to make treatment easy. Clients could call or text us on their way to work or during their lunch break. There were no observed drug tests into blue toilet bowl water, no mandatory pill counts. We gave them a collection of urine drug screens that they could take in the privacy of their own home and then hold up to their video screen after they resulted. I felt pride when we flipped together through their welcome packet, complete with cute illustrations that described how to calculate their own COWS score, a measurement usually reserved for nurses and doctors to use when judging the severity of someone's withdrawal, so they knew when to start their buprenorphine from the comfort of their own home. I loved hearing patients gush about how much better this experience was than prior treatment attempts. Quietly and modestly, we were offering a radical alternative to the standard addiction care offered at methadone clinics. And, because of a grant, we were able to provide free care to those who couldn't otherwise pay. We were democratizing treatment.

Within a few months, we had enough clients to leave the sad-child-illustration behind and move into our own space, complete with its own bathroom. In the spacious waiting room, we placed a fiddle leaf fig tree in one corner and a fridge full of seltzer water in the other. Mid-century modern couches flanked an oak coffee table, copies of *Dwell* magazine splayed across its surface.

Soon, our model started to attract attention, and the CEO of a well-respected corporate medical group invited us for a meeting. This medical group staffed emergency departments across the country, including one where I sometimes worked, and the CEO hoped we could find a way to work together. Many of his docs were hesitant to start buprenorphine in the ED because they did not have a reliable place to send their patients for continued addiction care. But if they had a virtual option that could be accessed by anyone, anywhere, that might be a different story.

Riding the elevator up to his office, I was rocketed from an hourly shift worker in the ED to the big leagues. Giddiness sneaked across our faces as my coworker and I sat in leather chairs across from the CEO, staring out his floor-length windows into San Francisco Bay. As we pitched why he should choose us to run their addiction services, he leaned forward and listened carefully. Suddenly, my opinion mattered.

After our meeting, we celebrated by scarfing down a wax-paper–lined bowl of nachos at a cheesy Tex-Mex restaurant down the block. Leaning in from the vinyl booth seats, we clinked our big plastic cups together in a toast. Although we were only drinking ice water, I felt buzzed all the same.

In contrast to the emergency department patients whom I only saw once before catapulting back into the world, I developed long-lasting relationships with my patients at the clinic. I know it sounds like a cheesy pharmaceutical ad when I say that bupe saved their lives, but it was true. One of my favorite patients was a young woman who had been addicted to pills. We often talked on her way to work as a veterinary assistant, video off so as not to distract her driving. I found myself uplifted by her skyward trajectory, as if her successes were my own. I gushed congratulations when she resolved all her court cases, when she excelled in her college courses, when she made breakthroughs in therapy, when she didn't relapse during a bad car accident. She had taken back her life.

But, also, I started to notice another pattern among my patients, both in the startup and the ED. At first, I assumed they were just a series of unrelated anomalies: when a pharmacist refused to fill my patient's prescription for buprenorphine because they lived in a different county than where I worked, or because I had prescribed buprenorphine from an emergency department and not a methadone clinic, or because the patient had filled opioid prescriptions early in the past—suggesting that they had the disease (opioid use disorder) that my prescribed medication was intended to treat. Certainly, one or two pharmacists might be risk-averse or misunderstand the regulations around buprenorphine prescribing.

But the more it happened, the more I realized that the problem extended beyond a handful of individual pharmacists. My patients already knew this, and were unfazed when such barriers appeared before them. They regularly experienced abnormally long wait times and received sideways glances when they tried to pick up their bupe at the pharmacy, or even flat-out verbal assault along the lines of "Look, we don't want any junkies around here."[5] Instead, they were surprised when the process was hassle-free.

Initially, I assumed this was stigma against people who used drugs, pure and simple. Later, I'd learn it was a little more complicated, as stigma itself had been baked into the web of arcane policies that shaped the treatment landscape, the DEA occasionally targeting pharmacies that dispensed "too much" buprenorphine.[6] Being cautious did not automatically mean someone held untoward views toward people with substance use, but, for several years, I would see the two as synonymous. Once I had seen the shadow of stigma, its apparition could no longer hide—it was everywhere. And once the medical board complaint arrived, I was further convinced that stigma was public enemy number one.

2019

Soft, unfiltered light streamed in through the old glass windows of the Craftsman house we rented, and a winter draft slipped in around the poorly insulated panes. As it was still morning, long shadows danced across the wooden floorboards. My first baby was due in less than a week, and I was trying to get my headspace ready to welcome a new life. I wanted to think less about work, more about fostering a welcoming presence. I grabbed my fleece coat and stepped into the damp air, carefully navigating my round body down the concrete steps and toward the mailbox.

Inside was a large manila envelope with a return address from Lansing, Michigan. As I trudged back up to the living room, I inspected the seal stamped upon the front, an eagle stretching its wings between a moose and an elk. I wasn't expecting any mail from Michigan, certainly nothing this official. My only connection to the state was the startup, as their headquarters was in Ann Arbor. I wondered if the envelope might contain an award, some formal recognition of how accessible we had made addiction treatment.

Eagerly, I ripped it open and held the stapled-together business letter in front of me, the bottom creases of the pages folding slightly upon my enormous belly. Much like text messages from my mom, the letterhead was in all caps, and the sender was none other than Michigan's Medical Board. It was definitely not an award. "Dear Licensee," it began. "Enclosed is an Administrative Complaint

(Complaint) charging you with violation(s) of the Public Health Code. You must respond to this Complaint IN WRITING WITHIN 30 DAYS from the day you received it. If you fail to do so, the Complaint will be sent to your Board's Disciplinary Subcommittee (DSC) to impose a sanction." Warmth rushed into my cheeks, and anxiety pulsed in my temples as the words deflated my state of peace. I was still not sure what I had done wrong after quickly scanning the first page, which simply explained that I could obtain legal representation before requesting a settlement or a formal hearing.

I flipped to the next page, and there, toward the bottom of the page, I found my first clue: "Suboxone is known as 'prison heroin,' and is commonly abused and diverted." Prison heroin? Really? Suboxone was increasingly seen as the gold standard treatment for opioid use disorder; it was not some fringe, illicit drug.[7] The language in the letter read less like one from an official medical board, which was supposed to be based in science, and more like propaganda from some abstinence-based troll on social media. Yet here it was. "From May 2018 through September 2018, Respondent wrote seventeen (17) prescriptions for controlled substances in Michigan. . . . Respondent's conduct constitutes a violation of general duty, consisting of negligence or failure to exercise due care, and fails to conform to minimal standards of acceptable, prevailing practice for the health profession."

Where once there had been a chorus of birds outside, now there was just a loud, monotonous buzzing inside my head. What did this mean? The legal jargon was confusing. What had I done wrong? What was at stake? Would I lose my medical license? The last four years of medical school, three years of residency, and one year of fellowship all made obsolete? How would I repay my $262,000 of student debt? My medical license, and thus my career, lay in the hands of the anonymous authorities behind this letter. The edges of my imagined future started to blur and swirl into formless colors, dissipating before my eyes.

I rested one hand on my belly, worried that my panic would cause labor to begin, and used the other to call Warren. The words tumbled out of my mouth—"administrative complaint," "medical board," "Michigan," "negligence," "prison heroin," "my license," "my job"—and I walked into the baby's nursery, which at this point, was no more than a cluttered guest room primarily used for storage. As I couldn't quite believe that a new little person would be joining our family, I had put off decorating her room. Although I did not want to be as eager as those pregnant women on social media who painted murals and hung matching arcs of tassels when they were still in their first trimester, now I wished I had at least done *something*. There wasn't even a place for me to sit in the room, and I craved a warm, fuzzy place to help ground me. My angst vibrated faster as I thought of all that still needed to be done, like assembling the crib and baby-proofing the house.

As we spoke, I stuffed a muumuu, slippers, and snacks into the empty hospital go-bag that lay in the corner. Even before I realized I was the subject of an investigation, uncertainty had buzzed through these final days of pregnancy; the baby could come at any moment. Now I felt completely unmoored. The potential impact of the investigation loomed large in my imagination. What if I could no longer practice medicine? I hoped that each item packed would help me wrestle some semblance of control over my life.

"Slow down. What happened?" Warren asked, the level of urgency rising in his voice. I pictured him running his fingers through his short, straight hair. He asked, "What does this mean for you, for us?" He had so many questions that I couldn't answer that I stopped trying to, instead reading portions of the letter aloud. Then he'd understand exactly what I knew and how much I didn't. Even without fully comprehending the content, it clearly sounded bad, very bad. I imagined him pacing at his office desk, hands on his hips, as he asked, "Wait, so you broke the law?"

According to the letter, I guess I had, one called "MCL 333.16221(a)," whatever that was. I started over on page 1, this time reading more slowly. They were going after me for a small technical error—a regulatory oversight and a few slips made by harried pharmacists. It seemed like something they would normally overlook. In fact, it was something they themselves had told us not to worry about.

A few months prior, one of our nurse practitioners at the Michigan clinic suddenly quit, affecting a handful of patients who needed their buprenorphine prescriptions refilled that week. If they didn't receive their prescriptions, we were worried they might relapse.

We asked our Chicago-based attorneys if I could write a few prescriptions for these patients, even though I had never seen them in person, as we were concerned that this might violate the stipulations of an in-person visit required by the Ryan Haight Act. Our attorneys assured us this would be fine; such temporary bridges were permitted. But it could only be temporary.

Not a problem—one prescription would buy us a few weeks, enough time for the patients to return to the clinic for an in-person visit with a new provider. As some of the affected patients lived in the Upper Peninsula, hours away from the Ann Arbor clinic, they couldn't drop everything to come for a visit within a few days. Understandably, they needed more notice.

But what our attorneys didn't know was that in Michigan, additional state licenses were required to prescribe opioids and buprenorphine: a Controlled Substance License and a Drug Treatment Program Prescriber License. Our company's attorneys had been selected for their experience with tech startups, not with healthcare. And because these licenses didn't exist in California, I didn't even know this was a requirement that could exist.

A few hours after I called in these patients' prescriptions, I tried to log in to Michigan's prescription monitoring program. Such programs had quickly become a staple part of each state's arsenal to fight the opioid epidemic. Before writing prescriptions for a controlled substance like a benzodiazepine or opioid, doctors were supposed to look up their patients in the online database and search for "suspicious" behavior: refilling medications too early, obtaining prescriptions from too many different providers, taking benzos and opioids together, or simply filling too many prescriptions for opioids. Such actions might suggest that a patient had developed addiction, was selling their pills, or was at risk of overdose, and thus we shouldn't prescribe any more. Although prescription drug monitoring programs had met their aim—physicians stopped prescribing as many pills—one could argue that they actually worsened the opioid epidemic, turning patients toward the black market. Graphs from this time period illustrated this dangerous trend quite strikingly: a blue line representing prescription misuse plummeted while a red line representing heroin soared.

I had never before visited Michigan's prescription monitoring website, as our medical assistants downloaded the info and placed it directly in the patients' charts. Furthermore, I didn't have any patients of my own in Michigan; I just supervised the nurse practitioners and physician assistants working there. But when I tried to log in to the database, I received an error message: To gain access, I first needed a Michigan Controlled Substance License. *A what?* I quickly typed the term into my browser's search bar. *Oh. Shit.* Panic pushed on my chest as I raced to call our COO. In turn, she called the pharmacies where I had sent prescriptions. She canceled the two that hadn't yet been filled, but for the other three, it was too late.

The next day, our attorneys anonymously called the Michigan Medical Board and asked if we needed to report such an error. "Oh, no," the board assured them. "Not for just three prescriptions. That's not the kind of person we would go after. And we don't really have a formal mechanism to report that. Furthermore, you are trying to do the right thing, calling us and all. So don't worry about it. We only go after the egregious docs." Relief quickly made me forget the entire incident. That was, until now. They saw me as a modern-day script doctor.

The original script doctors hailed from our country's first opioid epidemic in the nineteenth century. More than just a tale of a couple of rogue doctors, their story contained the origins of today's failed treatment landscape.

In 1863, it was estimated that 4 percent of the US population was addicted to opioids.[8] Part of the issue was cheap, easy access. Walk into any pharmacy, and you could buy syrups and salves containing opium, morphine, and codeine—no prescription needed. Did you have diarrhea? A cough? A headache? Was your baby teething? Did you have a drooping spirit? Try Winslow's Soothing Syrup, first marketed in 1849, a pleasant elixir of morphine and alcohol.[9]

It took decades for doctors to realize that such ingredients commonly added to over-the-counter medications could be habit-forming.[10] But, even if they had, there was no way to know where they were hiding. Until the 1906 Pure Food and Drug Act, medication labels didn't have to list their active ingredients, and drug companies were afraid that consumers would be scared off if they knew what they actually contained.

By the end of the nineteenth century, a constellation of factors had laid the groundwork for drug criminalization: the recognition of addictive substances, consumer annoyance with unregulated patent medicines, rising importation of opium, and plain old racism.

When an economic downturn hit San Francisco in the 1870s, white people blamed Chinese immigrants for stealing their jobs. In response, politicians began to villainize opium smoking, an activity associated with the Chinese community.[11] Newspaper headlines warned of the "Chinese Evil," "Chinese Invasion," and the "Opium Curse," and stories circulated about the power of opium to corrupt respectable white women into running off with Chinese men or becoming prostitutes.[12] Many whites even believed that the Chinese community was trying to hook them on opium in order to undermine American society.[13]

In response, the City of San Francisco passed our country's first antidrug legislation in 1875: an ordinance prohibiting the smoking of opium in "dens."[14] The city then tried to forcibly move everyone living in Chinatown into an area of the city reserved for pig farms.[15] When the courts ruled this policy as unconstitutional, the authorities turned to launching massive raids on Chinese homes and businesses in the name of eradicating opium. The confiscated material was thrown into a giant bonfire, and, as one observer described, "the choking smoke spread its heavy mantle over Chinatown like a pall upon the dead."[16]

Similarly, in the southeastern United States, it was racism against the Black community that garnered the momentum needed to prohibit drugs and criminalize addiction. Although influential whites such as Sigmund Freud and the former surgeon general of the US Army had publicly lauded the benefits of cocaine, the fear of the cocainized Black man coincided with the peak of lynching, legalized segregation, and restrictive voting laws.[17] White fear around cocaine provided just one more excuse as to why they could further target and police the Black community. Whites were afraid that, under the influence of cocaine, Black men would "become oblivious of their prescribed bounds and attack white society."[18] Many police departments at that time so believed that cocaine made African Americans impervious to standard bullets that they actually increased the caliber of their revolvers.[19]

This is exactly the same kind of inflammatory language used today when speaking about fentanyl and methamphetamine: Mexicans making fentanyl in illicit labs in the jungle, Mexicans sneaking drugs over the border—like there is some kind of boogeyman plotting to destroy us. Such exaggerated caricatures of good and evil seem like they belong more in my daughters' fairy-tale books than in journalism. This fable also implies that the solution involves building a bigger wall, deporting more immigrants, and prioritizing policing via "fentanyl homicide" laws and the criminalization of homelessness. For over one hundred years, white supremacy and the stigmatization of addiction have been inextricably linked, weaponizing drug panic to scapegoat, control, and persecute minoritized populations.

But even the DEA's own data will show you that such supply-focused approaches don't work. Despite a growing number of fentanyl seizures at the US-Mexico border every year, the number of fentanyl deaths continues to increase. Fentanyl is highly potent, cheaply manufactured, and easily snuck through ports of entry (or even produced within our own country). Additionally, opioid use disorder is much more common in America than in Mexico. Instead of blaming others, perhaps we should be directing our attention inward: Why do Americans like drugs so much?

By 1900, many states had already drafted their own anti-morphine laws.[20] Some restricted the sale of narcotics to doctors and pharmacists, and others prohibited opioid maintenance altogether, believing the only motivation to keep patients dependent on opioids was to enrich the doctors prescribing them. As most physicians believed that a patient would be forever cured once they made it through the throes of withdrawal, this approach made some sense. Additionally, many states thought strict punishments were necessary to motivate people to follow the law. There was no understanding of how addiction was a chronic disease marked by ongoing cravings and frequent relapse, how people would continue to use despite the risk of punishment.

In 1914, Congress passed the Harrison Act, effectively banning opioid maintenance for decades to come. Although this act has had a substantial legacy upon addiction treatment, at the time, it wasn't seen as a big deal. Unlike the Eighteenth Amendment, the Harrison Act did not position itself as a prohibition law; rather, it was simply a way to regulate and monitor the sale of opioids. It mandated that opioids could only be obtained via a prescription written by a licensed physician, and, thus, they could no longer be sold over the counter.[21] The act even had a clause asserting the right of a physician to prescribe opioids: "Nothing contained in this section shall apply . . . to the dispensing or distribution of any of the aforesaid drugs to a patient by a physician, dentist, or veterinary surgeon registered under this Act in the course of his professional practice only."[22] But that last clause, vague and open to interpretation, was the crux that ultimately transformed addiction care in the United States.

When the act came into effect in March 1915, and patients could no longer buy their opioids over the counter, they began to flood physicians' offices, forming long lines where before there had been none. Doctors were overwhelmed; there was no way they could adequately treat this many new patients, let alone the ones they already had—nor did they want to. There were reports of violence attributed to desperate attempts to obtain drugs and the delirious state of sudden withdrawal.[23] In New York City, the cost of heroin on the street rose from $6.50 an ounce to about $100.[24] Drug-related arrests for possession skyrocketed, quickly crowding court calendars. Before addiction was criminalized, it was not a big problem. Now it was.

The medical community was divided on how to respond. Was addiction treatable? Was there a cure? They didn't even know if withdrawal itself could be deadly. Some physicians prescribed tapered courses of opioids for withdrawal, either in the monitored setting of a hospital detox or at home. Others recommended cold turkey as the best approach. Only a minority believed that long-term maintenance with opioids was needed for those who had failed attempts at abstinence, especially if maintenance enabled a fairly normal life.

However, those outside the medical community did not recognize such nuances. By and large, they did not think there was any reason to dispense opioids to people with dependence. Because the Harrison Act was just a tax act, its enforcement fell to the Bureau of Internal Revenue within the Treasury Department. Almost overnight, revenue agents started to warn and arrest physicians and pharmacists who provided opioids to addicts or prescribed what they considered to be "excessive amounts." Their enforcement was confusing to many in the medical community, as the revenue agents were neither physicians nor attorneys—how were they the ones able to determine what amounts of opioids were appropriate?[25] When cases were brought to court, the burden of proof was placed upon the defendant, and even those who escaped conviction had their careers ruined by the publicity.[26]

In response, the majority of physicians stopped prescribing opioids. They weren't sure what was allowed and what wasn't. Furthermore, most doctors had no interest in treating people who used drugs, sharing the prevailing view that addicts were untrustworthy.[27] A small percentage of physicians continued to prescribe opioids, believing that there was nothing in the Harrison Act that explicitly forbade them from doing so. Generally, these doctors fell into two camps: those who prescribed because they believed that maintenance was the best treatment for addiction, and those who prescribed to make a profit.[28]

The latter were pejoratively referred to as "script doctors," and Dr. Webb of Memphis, Tennessee, was one of the most notorious.[29] Running his fingers through his beard, he would listen as patients described how they couldn't stop, how they had to keep using more to simply feel normal. "Do you want a prescription?" he would ask, already knowing the answer. Patients didn't come to him for anything else; some patients even drove hundreds of miles to see him. When they'd nod their head yes, eagerness in their eyes, he'd ask the follow-up question: "Do you have fifty cents?" Money was withdrawn, a prescription was signed, and an exchange was made. If the patient had more money, more prescriptions were provided, each with a different name. According to Supreme Court recordings, Webb sold over four thousand prescriptions.[30] This was likely how the Michigan Medical Board perceived me, even though I had only prescribed buprenorphine to five patients.

Prominent physicians wrote op-eds criticizing such script doctors. The New York Health Commissioner, Dr. Royal S. Copeland, said that physicians who sold prescriptions to addicts "should be boiled in oil."[31] The government listened.[32] Webb's case made it all the way to the Supreme Court, whose members did not distinguish between legitimate maintenance and willy-nilly prescribing. In 1919, the court declared that maintenance treatment, in its intent to keep addicts comfortable, was not "in the course of professional treatment," as it did not offer a "cure."[33] Abstinence had officially won.

Once the *Webb* decision was made, the raids on physicians and pharmacists began. Of the 81,000 physicians practicing in New York City at the time, less than 40 continued to prescribe narcotics for those with addiction.[34] The bureau subsequently indicted them all for "trafficking in drugs." Addiction had become a crime, and patients, physicians, and pharmacists were all considered suspects. Marie wrote, "Overnight a million victims of a horrifying illness were transformed into criminals."[35]

In 1981, David Courtwright asked Marie, "Which groups would you identify as the most influential opponents of methadone maintenance?" She answered, "My feeling was always that the Narcotic Bureau that turned the doctors against addicts, that scared them out of the treatment. . . . As far as I like to think of it, the Narcotics men had really so scared the doctors that they abandoned the treatment of drug addiction, and therefore, there is no place for them to go. So they would be against addicts in the sense that professionally, they are denying a group of people treatment."[36]

Once I knew this history, I began to see the Michigan Medical Board investigation in a new context. The board was simply continuing the century-long tradition of criminalizing maintenance medications and the doctors who prescribed them. Even though addiction docs such as myself were reducing the demand for illegal opioids, enforcement saw our contribution to the opioid supply as the graver offense. Via telemedicine, I was making buprenorphine too accessible. Although changes in federal regulation meant that agents could no longer straight-out arrest doctors like me who prescribed medications for opioid use disorder, they could still get us when we broke small technicalities, an error easy to make in today's confusing regulatory patchwork.

Such an approach framed a systemic problem—stigma against addiction treatment—as an individual failing: a doctor who was too loose with her prescription pad, that is, a modern-day script doctor. The goal? To scare doctors away from offering addiction treatment. They had also tried this with Marie. And, by and large, it worked.

After I got off the phone with Warren, I called our COO, who promised to call our attorneys and set up a meeting within a few hours. While I waited, I reached out to others who I hoped might support me. Since Andrew Herring had been doing similar work for several years now, pioneering the way forward and emboldening us to follow suit, I figured he would have heard of similar cases, or maybe even experienced such a case himself. Maybe he knew some harm reduction attorneys who could offer advice.

He quickly texted me back, saying he would call one of the directors at the California Health Care Foundation and a colleague who used to work in Michigan. But, unfortunately, neither of those connections led to anything. They didn't know me; this wasn't their problem. Besides, I'm sure they were dealing with more pressing issues. I also emailed the president of the Michigan chapter of the American Society of Addiction Medicine. Myself a member, I assumed they would be outraged that the medical board referred to buprenorphine as prison heroin. Who knew how many other doctors had been accused of the same thing? Once ASAM heard of this, surely they would start advocating to change the medical board's opinion.

Instead, the president emailed back to recuse herself from discussing my situation, as she herself was on the Michigan Medical Board. Were addiction doctors themselves leading the charge against treatment? Later, I'd learn that Marie and Vince felt the same betrayal, and were outraged by the medical community's silence when regulators circumscribed their ability to offer effective treatment. A cruel loneliness settled into my bones; there was nobody to help shoulder the repercussions or to help guide me through this experience. If only I had a mentor, someone to help me forge this path through the wilderness. But, like Marie, I was doing this alone. Maybe she could become the guiding star I was searching for.

When Warren arrived home from work, he immediately came to find me. I was in the kitchen, throwing dinner together before running off to my poetry class that evening, the aroma of butter sizzling around me. Although nightfall came early in January, the window shades were still up, my daily attempt to harness more light from Northern California's temperate climate. Our house was at the bottom of a redwood forest that thrived on a year-round supply of mist and clouds. On nights like these, I especially missed the desert sun. "Any news?" he asked as he wrapped his arms around me. We were exactly the same height, and, when I wasn't pregnant, we were also the same size. I rested my cheek against his soft flannel shirt.

"Yeah, the legal team is going to help," I responded, pulling away from his embrace to grab more vegetables out of the fridge. I rattled off the steps the attorneys had suggested; fixating on their plan helped my anxious mind ignore the real issue at hand—that this investigative action would leave a permanent mark on my record, something I would have to explain every time I applied for a new job, renewed my medical license, or moved to a new state.

Warren's words rushed out: "Could your hospital make you take an administrative leave? Could the California Medical Board refuse to renew your license? Would that mean that you couldn't work as a doctor anymore?" Warren was the more rule-abiding member of our partnership. Although he was a scientific analyst who modeled drought scenarios for municipal water districts, he had learned the world of medicine through the years at my side. He reached into the fridge for a beer, and I extended my hand to take a swig before returning the can to his palm. One sip wouldn't hurt the baby this close to her due date, but this level of panic might.

"I don't know." I shrugged. "That's what I'm worried about, too." Of all the doomsday scenarios, the most likely seemed that my hospital might tell me not to return to work until all of this was resolved, which could take months. We were also contemplating moving back to Arizona, and I worried that this "disciplinary action" could sabotage all our dreams. For the last couple of years, my work in emergency medicine had left me exhausted and burned out. Tired of working shifts across the Bay Area, I decided to accept a full-time position as the medical director and chair of an emergency department in Alameda. I hoped this new role might offer a professional home and lessen my burnout, as an "upward" move might feel a little less like floundering. Instead, it brought new stresses, leaving me desperate for a way out. Also, I wanted to raise our daughter under the wild, open skies I loved, not in the middle of an urban metropolis where everyone was fighting to survive or get ahead. The very next day, I had an informal call scheduled with an acquaintance at the University of Arizona.

Warren's forehead creased, and the volume of his voice raised. "This is what happens when working for a startup. They don't know what they are doing. They let this happen to you, but now it's you who is being punished." I cocked an eyebrow and nodded; he wasn't wrong. Startups were notorious for skirting the rules, which was part of their appeal. When governments took too long to respond to a problem, an innovative company could zip in and cobble together a solution. Yet I was the only one in the company's leadership with a medical license to lose. Warren asked, "Are you going to quit?"

I vigorously shook my head. "No, the work we are doing is too important." That was the one thing I was still sure of. Additionally, I liked the job—it was fun to shape a medical company, and I liked the creative challenge that came with being a CMO.

He sighed with exasperation.

"I don't want to think about this anymore. I have to leave for class." I ladled some curry into my bowl, slung my purse over my shoulder, and waddled out to the car.

Two nights a week, I took classes at Mills, a historically women's college whose campus was peppered with towering eucalyptus and verdant lush lawns. Following the advice of one of my mentors at the health department, I was pursuing a master of fine arts in creative writing. I wasn't sure how the arts might help my career, but that wasn't the point. Writing offered me a path toward deeper understanding, a way to shape the random events of daily life into a meaningful arc. Although medicine brought me face-to-face with life and death, it couldn't help me make sense of it. The arts could.

That night was my first poetry class of the semester, held in the third story of Mills Hall, a white wooden building built in the 1800s and buttressed by columns. I walked past a chorus of frogs in the nearby stream, creaked my way up the wooden staircase, and took a seat by the open window, too ancient to have a screen. Our class was small, around ten students, and taught by Truong Tran, a gregarious professor whom the poets unanimously adored. That night, he picked up a piece of chalk and scribbled on the board, "What haunts us? What hunts us? What are we hunting?" At the time, I wasn't sure; I didn't yet understand the impact the day's events would have in the years to come, nor the role of addiction or writing. After a brief pause, Truong instructed, "The answer to that is our life's work."

Less than a week after receiving the complaint, I gave birth to a chunky little girl weighing almost nine pounds, Finley. The labor had been long—almost thirty hours—yet almost immediately after her arrival, I was already back on the phone with our attorney. I shifted my weight in the stiff hospital bed, trying unsuccessfully to find a more comfortable position. A plastic incontinence sheet stuck to my thighs and an overnight pad affixed to the disposable mesh underwear wedged between my legs, I cradled my baby across my chest with one arm, her floppy body trying to adjust to this new world, and held my phone in the other. This was not the scene that Warren and I had envisioned during our labor and delivery classes.

I spoke into the phone's speaker: "Do I need to buy a plane ticket to Michigan?"

"No, we can arrange a phone conference instead. It shouldn't make much of a difference."

"What are the next steps?" I asked, starting to rock my torso back and forth as Finley yawned, reminding me of my own fatigue.

"I'll draft a letter on your behalf, showing how you are an exemplary physician. You're the opposite of negligent."

"Okay, I can send you my CV. Will that help? It shows that I'm a member of ASAM, I've given lectures on buprenorphine, I'm an attending at a residency program, and more recently I've become the medical director of an emergency department. Is that helpful?"

"Yeah, that will all be great."

"Do you think they'll drop the complaint?" The baby sighed as her eyes flickered shut. Her cheek twitched slightly.

"No. There is no way. They're pretty strict about this stuff. But I'd like to negotiate with them, offering to pay a higher fee in exchange for them downgrading the severity of their charge from an act of negligence to a fine."

So that's what this was about for them—money. It felt like something so much larger for me. But, still, I was relieved. A "fine" sounded much better than a "negligent act." I closed my eyes and leaned back. "So, what does that mean?"

"No matter what happens, this will forever be listed as a disciplinary action in the National Provider Data Bank. It will be part of the public record, and you'll have to report it every time you apply for a new job or renew your medical license."

My mouth felt as dry as the desert. I reached over the side rail for a sip of ice water from the Styrofoam cup resting on the roller table. For the rest of my life, this would be something to be explained. At the very least, it would lengthen the application process at various hospitals and state medical boards, as an official committee would need to review my records. At worst, it would affect my chance to work at individual hospitals or within specific states. As I had never gone through this, nor knew anybody who had, I wasn't exactly sure how it would affect me. Soon, I would also learn that it hindered our ability to refinance my student loans and obtain a mortgage. My first few days of motherhood, ones saturated by the doughy vulnerability that comes with sleep deprivation, plummeting hormones, and baby cuddles, would also be filled with anxiety.

CHAPTER 4

Narco

1946–1947

Like me, Marie never thought she would become an addiction physician. When she graduated from medical school in 1944, she planned to pursue orthopedic surgery. But instead of going straight to residency after her internship, she joined many of her classmates in the fight against Hitler. She enlisted in the US Navy, believing she would serve as an orthopedic surgeon and oversee a fifty-bed hospital in China.[1] But the navy had no use for women doctors, or, as Marie put it, "They didn't really have a uniform for me," so she was sent to the US Public Health Service (USPHS) Narcotic Farm in Lexington, Kentucky, where she would work as an addiction psychiatrist.[2]

For a New Yorker who had her sights set on serving abroad and becoming an orthopedist, I cannot think of a more diametric fate. I would have been heartbroken as I watched my future completely evaporate, powerless to dictate the course of my life. But, in her subsequent interviews, Marie laughed and breezed through this anecdote of foregone dreams.

Instead, she claimed it was she who changed her mind about surgery, all on her own. She told Courtwright, "I didn't see myself as a good surgeon. I love being the first assistant to surgery, I love being the surgeon's assistant so to speak, but not the main surgeon. . . . I don't think I quite had the temperament for surgery. I want more closeness with the patient rather than with his kidney or gallbladder."

But I don't believe her. Her explanation feels like a reshaping of the narrative, wrestling a storyline that was outside of her control and forging it into one that she herself designed. She was a talented pianist, skilled with her hands; surely this dexterity would have transferred beautifully to the embodied practice of surgery.

Additionally, when she provided this justification to Courtwright, she was already a famous addiction physician well aware of the pivotal role that Lexington served in her career: It was her introduction to methadone, to addiction, to the field that made her famous. When gazed at from a successful future, painful events took on a positive sheen. But how did she feel at the moment her post was switched, the moment she realized she would no longer become a surgeon? All she could see was what had been lost, not the better future that would eventually fill the space.

I also wonder if a lack of female role models contributed to her reluctance to be the "main surgeon." Today, orthopedic surgery is one of the most male-dominated specialties, if not the most, with almost 85 percent of its residents being men.[3] In contrast, psychiatry was a field more welcoming to women during Marie's time. As Marie said during an interview with Sarah Lawrence's alumni magazine, "Psychiatry is an ideal profession for a married woman—you can arrange your own hours and still keep up a practice at home. It is one profession where, for the most part, a woman is more tolerated than a man."[4]

Driving west from Lexington, the stone and brick buildings of Narco first appeared as tiny dots on the crest of a distant hill. Narco sat on 1,200 acres of rolling Kentucky bluegrass, the landscape so empty that Marie could see the exact point where the expansive sky met the bright green fields stretching in all directions. With anticipation, she crossed her legs in the back seat and leaned forward to catch a better view. She wore pumps and a simple dress that reached her shins. As she rolled down her window, she felt the moisture in the air and heard the buzz of cicadas. When her driver turned down the road that led to the prison, a guard in a little brick station stepped out. He was in the middle of rolling a cigarette when he paused to wave them by. At least, this is how I imagine it.

The Lexington Narcotic Farm opened in 1935, costing $4 million and three years to construct.[5] Its mission was threefold: to incarcerate, rehabilitate, and study people addicted to drugs. After the 1914 Harrison Act effectively criminalized addiction, people who used drugs began crowding federal prisons, sneaking drugs inside and introducing them to incarcerated people who had never before used, and became somewhat of a problem for the wardens.[6] In response, wardens lobbied for the establishment of a prison solely for addicts, and progressives lobbied for hospitals to treat addiction. As a compromise, Congress passed an act creating two narcotic farms, one in Lexington, Kentucky, and the other in Fort Worth, Texas, jointly managed by the Public Health Service and the Bureau of Prisons. From the beginning, the United States could not decide whether addiction was a disease or a crime.

Only once Marie neared the main complex could she fully grasp its enormity. In the distance, silos and dairy barns stood alongside the tomato crops, and black-and-white cows rested lazily in the clover. A red tractor idled in the foreground as two shirtless men heaved the remaining bales of hay onto a truck bed. At any one point, the farm could have as many as eight hundred pigs and one hundred beef cows, providing almost all the meat consumed in the institution. As it was believed that a healthy relationship to work could override a user's desire to use drugs, patients cared for livestock, harvested the fields, and worked as blacksmiths. Additionally, patient labor kept the institution running.

The entrance was the most impressive building of all, its central tower flanked by four-story columns and topped with a teal triangular prism. It was designed to resemble a temple, one of rehabilitation. Marie's driver parked the car and led her up the short flight of white steps, where they waited under a towering arch for another guard to unlock the iron gate. Inside, the cavernous entrance hall was decorated by lofty vaulted ceilings, stylized silver light fixtures, and ornate Art Deco archways. Next to the guard's desk was a thin man with shaggy brown hair and pale skin standing patiently, suitcase in hand.

An orderly clacked down the hallway to the man, clipboard in hand. As their voices echoed off the high ceilings and cold floors, Marie surmised that the man was checking himself in. He had run out of heroin, and the chills, pain, and nausea of withdrawal had begun. Patients or incarcerated people—I am unsure of what to call them—either arrived voluntarily or at the behest of a judge. If it were the former, they were referred to as volunteers or "vols." Regardless, their intake was the same: they were strip-searched for paraphernalia and drugs, provided with uniforms, and then shuttled to the medical ward for a physical. As most hospitals refused to care for people with addiction, many of Narco's arrivals had untreated diseases like tuberculosis.

Then patients went to detox, where they received gradually decreasing doses of morphine (and, later, methadone) until they were withdrawn completely from opioids. In contrast to the jails that offered nothing, Narco's medicated detox was quite compassionate.[7] After about two weeks in detox, patients were transferred to the general population, where all further treatment was abstinence-based.

That was when the majority of the vols checked out, more interested in the temporary comfort of medications than in sobriety. In his autobiographical novel *Junky*, William S. Burroughs describes such a scenario: "You are allowed seven days to rest in population after medication stops. Then you have to choose a job and go to work. . . . I did not figure to stay around long enough to work."[8]

Staff did not appreciate this. How could their patients achieve sobriety if they left before the real treatment even began? They did not come to work every day just to offer a temporary respite for people who were out of heroin; they came to offer a lasting cure. So, in 1946, Kentucky legislators passed a law classifying habitual narcotic use—addiction—as a misdemeanor punishable with up to one year in jail. Then, if a patient tried to leave early, staff called the sheriff, who effectively prevented them from leaving until the doctor said they were done.[9] Once again, the lines were blurred between patient and inmate, healthcare provider and law enforcer.

Even today, many people believe that compulsory addiction treatment is in a user's best interest, that the harms incurred by taking away someone's autonomy are justified if sobriety is the end result.

Many states are actively passing and expanding laws that allow parents, police, or concerned others to petition courts to force users into rehab.[10] But the data suggests that these coercive approaches don't work, with the majority of people returning to drug use as soon as they are discharged.[11] Worse than that, these approaches might actually increase someone's risk of fatal overdose.[12]

But, at Narco, Kentucky's legislation did little to scare away new patients. Narco often housed 1,000 to 1,500 patients at a time, and the majority were volunteers.[13] Narco's therapeutic model was predicated upon four distinct elements: medicated drug withdrawal, residence in a drug-free environment, psychotherapy, and supervised activities including recreation and "therapeutic labor."[14] There were bowling alleys, softball fields, and tennis courts. As William Burroughs Jr. put it, "It was a country club, as prisons go."[15] Men from the city learned how to milk cows and grow kale, even though these skills would not be particularly useful when they returned home. But, even with such a robust program, the relapse rate of former Narco patients hovered around 90 percent.[16]

Many argued that the relapse rate was so high because patients had no addiction services when they returned to their communities, nor would anybody hire a former user or convict. Even today, many people with a criminal record have difficulty returning to life as a "normal" citizen because the right to vote, public benefits, employment, and housing are often taken away after incarceration.[17] Thus, Narco's alumni had nothing to do but return to old habits. Narco is a poignant reminder that compulsory abstinence-based treatment and incarceration are not going to solve our country's opioid epidemic—they never have. Yet we keep on trying.

From 1970 to 2010, the US penal population ballooned from 300,000 to more than 2 million, with drug convictions accounting for the majority of the increase.[18] Thanks to the war on drugs, the United States has one of the highest rates of incarceration in the world despite our below-average rate of crime.[19] And, as we have historically used drug arrests as a way to persecute minoritized populations, the impact of this war has fallen disproportionally on Black Americans. Even though people of all races use and sell illegal drugs at similar rates, Black people are much more likely to be incarcerated.[20] In some states, Black men are incarcerated at rates twenty to fifty times those of white men for drug charges.[21] Yet, despite all these arrests, our country's opioid epidemic has only worsened. In 2001, there were an estimated 9,496 opioid overdose deaths.[22] By 2022, that figure had climbed to 84,181.[23]

When Marie arrived at Narco, I wonder who first greeted her in that aspirational entrance hall with its arched ceilings and stunning architecture. Was it a nurse? Another US Public Health Service recruit? Let's say it was Dr. Harris Isbell, the recently appointed director of Narco's Addiction Research Center, and let's imagine that he took her on a tour of the facilities. As they walked down long gray corridors, Marie's eyes drifted from his slicked-back hair to the circular key ring hanging from his belt, upon which dangled twenty to thirty skeleton keys. As he unlocked gate after gate, the sense that she was in a prison, not a hospital, started to sink in. Patients began to take interest in this young woman, their leering eyes making her feel slightly uncomfortable. Although there were also female patients, they were segregated in a different ward. As Marie later told David Courtwright, "The patients were hardly anything to be desired because people in prison, including myself, are transformed into something other than what you are on the outside."

They walked by intake, where the young man from the lobby was now sitting in a chair in front of a large light, having his photo taken. A mug shot? They then walked past detox, where seven men were standing in line, all wearing the same wrinkled white pants and long-sleeved shirts, waiting expectantly for their shots of morphine.[24] Within a few months, the morphine would be replaced with methadone. In another room, nurses with crisp white aprons and caps clipped the nails of inmates; manicures and pedicures were considered a part of "the cure." As they entered the dayroom, the smell of cigarettes hung thick in the air. Marie, herself a heavy smoker, asked if they had time to stop for a smoke, too. Overhearing Marie's request, a patient playing cards at a large central table enthusiastically invited her over, but Dr. Isbell quickly ushered her away.

It was then that Marie first heard jazz music echoing down the hallway. Inside one of Narco's many practice rooms, a handful of patients were playing drums, a stand-up bass, a trumpet, and a piano. During Marie's year at Narco, she would often play piano alongside her patients, but not today. Dr. Isbell explained that they were practicing for this weekend's performance, leading her toward the 1,300-seat theater, complete with a velvet curtain draped across its stage.

Patients, staff, and even Lexington locals came to watch world-class jazz in the middle of rural Kentucky, but, once the band got going, it was hard to hear the music over all the yelling, whistling, and cheering from the crowd.[25] Chet Baker, Elvin Jones, Stan Levey, Jackie McLean, Red Rodney, Sonny Rollins, and many other famous jazz musicians all did time at Narco.[26] In New York, Narco was spoken of as if it were an elite jazz workshop, and some musicians even lied about having a heroin habit just so they could check in and study from the greats. When I shared this bit of information with my husband, he excitedly put together a Narco jazz playlist for us to listen to. As the fast drums of bebop raced along, I could almost imagine myself by Marie's side.

In the 1950s, it was estimated that 40 percent of jazz musicians used heroin—Billie Holiday and Charlie Parker being two of the most notorious.[27] As jazz was an avant-garde, multicultural blend of improvisations, polyrhythms, and harmonies associated with hip counterculture, prohibition speakeasies frequently invited jazz musicians to perform. Once heroin became a part of this subculture, jazz and addiction became inextricably linked. Users increasingly came from Black and Puerto Rican communities in New York, Chicago, Los Angeles, and Detroit, enclaves that had never before seen the harms that heroin could cause.

Harry Anslinger, the racist commissioner of the Federal Bureau of Narcotics from 1930 to 1962, hated jazz, likening it to "jungles in the dead of night" and the "unbelievable ancient indecent rites of the East Indies." He told his agents to specifically target jazz artists and "shoot first" in their drug raids, as jazz represented everything he hated: nonconformity, Blackness, and drugs.[28]

Anslinger is often considered the orchestrator of America's war on drugs, successfully drumming up hysteria around reefer madness and support for harsher drug sentencing. He once said, "The answer to the problem is simple—get rid of drugs, pushers, and users. Period."[29] In the face of today's easily synthesized fentanyl, such an approach seems not only naive, but impossible. Additionally, the majority of dealers are not mafiosos but regular people who have no other way to fund their addiction. By locking them up, we are effectively criminalizing their disease. But, by and large, the public supported Anslinger, as he linked crime, race, and drugs in a way that responded perfectly to the racist fears simmering within white America.[30] And they still do.

Now let's say that Dr. Isbell led Marie outside and toward a three-story brick building with a large tree shading its front steps[31]—the Addiction Research Center.[32] Narco wasn't there just to incarcerate and rehabilitate, but also to study addiction itself, and it was the ARC where such experiments occurred.

As they walked through the lab, the barking and whining of dogs grew louder and louder. Marie peered through an open doorway on their right, into a room lined with cages of dogs whose sad eyes pleaded with her. One even stood up, paws on the grate, hopeful that she might set him free. On the ground in front of them was a man who appeared to be a scientist, wearing a white lab coat and kneeling on the ground, using one hand to lift the nape of the dog's neck and the other to inject a clear solution from a glass hypodermic needle.

Dr. Isbell stopped to explain. "This is one of our patients working in the lab. We are testing to see whether or not methadon is addictive."[33]

Methadone was first synthesized in Germany around 1937 by Hoechst, a company with three hundred manufacturing plants and over twelve thousand workers.[34] Hoechst eventually became a part of I. G. Farben, a notorious conglomerate that included all of Germany's major pharmaceutical industries and played a leading role in numerous criminal activities and human rights violations under the Nazi regime. During World War II, they recruited subjects for drug trials from concentration camps, used slave labor, and developed nerve agents used in chemical warfare.[35] All of these activities were exposed during the Nuremberg trials, in which the director of Hoechst and many other scientists were indicted as war criminals.[36]

It is unclear if methadone was tested on prisoners in concentration camps, but it certainly seems possible. Human trials of methadone began during the height of the war in 1942, but all the records have since "disappeared." After the war ended in 1945, I. G. Farben was disbanded, and all its property, including its patents and records, was confiscated. Hoechst was placed under US military control, and a four-man team, including a chemist at pharmaceutical giant Eli Lilly, interviewed key Hoechst scientists, reviewed their research, and brought home drug samples and documents.

As methadone was of particular interest to them, only a few months passed before Eli Lilly successfully synthesized the drug in their own lab and began safety trials. After the FDA approved its use in 1947, Eli Lilly began to market the medication—which they called "methadon" and Dolophine—as a nonaddictive analgesic that treated pain two times better than morphine and for more than twice as long. Rightfully distrustful of the pharmaceutical company's claims, the ARC scientists began to conduct their own research—on patients.[37]

During this time in history, it was common practice to experiment on prisoners. It wouldn't be until the 1949 passage of the Nuremberg Code, a document that was developed in response to the Nazis' abusive human experimentation, that any policy would be developed to protect human research subjects.[38] The code dictated that human research subjects must have the capacity to give consent, exercise free choice, and have enough understanding to make an informed decision. However, even after the passage of the code, prisoners in the United States continued to be used as research subjects. When organizations spoke out against such practices, noting that prisoners could not fully consent because of the power differentials and coercion inherent in a prison setting, nothing really changed. In 1952, the American Medical Association, the foremost medical society in the United States, issued a resolution, "Disapproval of Participation in Scientific Experiments by Inmates of Penal Institutions," and mailed it to governors, state and federal prison officials, and parole boards.[39] But, without an enforcement mechanism, the resolution had no teeth, and so the research continued.

As if the link between methadone, Nazis, and prison research weren't sinister enough, there was also a connection to one of our country's most horrific medical experiments. The ARC was run under the auspices of the US Public Health Service, the same organization that was concurrently overseeing the Tuskegee Syphilis Study. In Tuskegee, scientists wanted to study the ways in which the syphilis spirochete wreaked havoc on the human body, starting first with a painless sore that disappeared in a few weeks, moving then to an infectious rash on the palms of the hands for a couple of months, and, eventually, to infecting the brain itself. Investigators enrolled about six hundred Black men, some with syphilis and some without, into their study, and promised free healthcare as a perk of enrollment. Yet the investigators never informed the men of their syphilis diagnoses or offered the simple cure—a shot of penicillin. When the forty-year study finally came to a halt in the 1970s, many of the patients had needlessly died from syphilis and its complications, their wives had been infected, and their children were born with congenital defects. Researchers saw the lives of Black patients as dispensable, their deaths justifiable in the name of science. Based on these atrocities, is it really so surprising that many leaders in the Black community distrusted methadone when it first came out in the 1960s and '70s?

When the Associated Press reporter Jean Heller broke the Tuskegee story in 1972, the medical establishment and country were left reeling.[40] How could health professionals, scientists, and the government—people who we trusted to care for us—allow such an atrocity to occur? In response, Congress opened an investigation into the US Public Health Service that would expose some of the ARC's questionable practices, including their covertly funded LSD research.[41]

But during Marie's stint at Narco, none of that had happened yet. Narco scientists saw drug users as the perfect subjects and a locked environment as the perfect setting. Dr. William Martin, the ARC research director from 1963 to 1977, explained, "From their practical experience they have much more knowledge about what the drugs will do than most other subjects and they understand much of the pharmacologic jargon."[42] And, as many of the patients lived in dorms at the ARC, follow-up was easy and guaranteed.[43]

As an incentive for patients to "volunteer" in drug trials, they were often "paid" in the drug of their choosing, whether it be heroin or cannabis. In one video from the ARC, two Black patients are rolling joints upon a wooden desk while a white physician sits across from them.[44] The camera focuses on the patient with buzzed hair and a white button-down shirt taking a hit, smoke streaming from the end of his thin paper cigarette. He then asks the patient at his side, a mustached man wearing a sweater with an orange and yellow pattern, "Have another one?"

He smiles and laughs. "Sure, why not, the government's paying for it."

The video then cuts to some of the experiments performed after the men were sufficiently high, the man in the white shirt spinning in a chair with electrodes taped to his face while a different patient lies on a bed with what appears to be a helmet made of white tape affixed to his scalp.

Many patients said they liked participating in the ARC trials, as they received both free drugs and a sense of purpose. It made them feel like they were a part of something bigger, like their addiction could help others. But, understandably, not everyone was so positive. Former test subject Eddie Flowers said, "Later on I came to grips with the fact that I was used. Being a young man, I was very vulnerable in the sense that if it's about drugs, I want drugs."[45]

Although Narco was complicit in human rights abuses, it is also responsible for the majority of what we know today about addiction and its treatment. In 1948, the first large-scale US trial of methadone involved 115 men at Lexington, all of whom had been addicted to morphine.[46] In 1951, Dr. Isbell and Dr. Abraham Wikler studied naloxone's prototype, Nalline, on twelve Narco patients with opioid use disorder.[47] In the 1970s, buprenorphine was pioneered by Dr. D. R. Jasinki. The ARC also created an objective way to assess opioid withdrawal, the precursor to today's COWS score. Before Narco, many physicians mistakenly believed that withdrawal symptoms were purely "hysterical" in origin.[48]

Dr. Isbell and the other researchers at the ARC were right about methadone—it did cause dependence—and in 1947, they published their results.[49] They also began to use methadone in their standard detox protocol instead of morphine, which would become Marie's first introduction to methadone.[50] When a patient arrived addicted to heroin, Marie would carefully switch him over to methadone, gradually decreasing the dose over the course of two weeks until he was no longer on any opioids at all.[51]

Today, this procedure is known as "medicated detox," and it is quite a different approach than methadone maintenance, where a patient receives methadone every single day, potentially for their entire life. Marie later wrote of medicated detox, "It is simple enough to withdraw a drug addict from drugs. Unfortunately, too much emphasis has been placed on the importance of this part of the therapy. Removing a patient from drugs and leaving him in a drug-free environment even for four months is not enough. A majority of the patients I have seen give a history of relapsing to the use of drugs within one to twenty-four hours upon release from an institution."[52] Because of this reality, most addiction experts today recommend methadone maintenance for years before tapering off.

After Marie and Dr. Isbell's tour of the ARC, they stepped into an idling car; it was time for Marie to settle into the space that would be her home for the next year. About half a mile down the road from the prison, they passed a large white mansion on top of a hill where patients gardened a terraced lawn. "That's where the Medical Officer in Charge lives," explained Dr. Isbell. Then they passed the other physician houses: two duplexes, a large white-washed house, a narrow red-brick home, and an apartment building for the doctors who weren't yet lugging families along.[53] But Marie would not be staying in those. As the only female physician,[54] she was instead relegated to a room in the nurses' house, a situation she would later describe as a "disaster," not because of the obvious gender inequality, which Marie seemed to gloss over, but because of the nurses' racism.[55]

When some of the nurses noticed Marie treating the patients with respect, they called her an "addict-lover" and several painfully racist names I won't repeat.[56] But because she not only worked with them but lived with them, too, she had no reprieve. Marie told Courtwright, "The nurses were old time nurses who had been in the public health service and worked in that prison for God knows how many years. . . . It was pretty rough, pretty rough for a little girl out of her internship"—she paused to laugh incongruously—"and who had no idea that people like this existed."[57]

As the days went on, she became more and more incensed by the staff's treatment of patients. She told Courtwright, "Prison attracts what precipitates out as a kind of bureaucrat, or a kind of personality that thrives on having prisoners work for them, or carrying around large collections of keys. Speaking to people harshly, autocratically, business, self-centered, meanwhile indulgent in themselves because their houses were manned by a group of prisoners who acted as servants in every capacity." She paused momentarily before continuing, "That was difficult."

On Sunday mornings, her commanding officer ordered her to join him for horseback rides because he wanted company. Marie said, "All I could think of was how appalling it was—how like being lord and lady of the manor—to go bounding over the prison grounds while the patients watched behind bars."[58]

Although she had no "particular interest in the addicts," she immersed herself in work, perhaps her own kind of escape. The hardest part of her job was performing parole evaluations, declaring whether or not a patient was eligible to leave Narco. Because she herself felt so claustrophobic in the locked wards, she couldn't imagine condemning another human being to further containment. Marie said, "It was horrible—being in a position to say when another human being is going to get in the sun again. I couldn't think of anything that would make me say 'no,' and I never did."

One day, she was caring for some women patients when she discovered that some of them hadn't left the women's quarters in four years, except for an occasional movie in the men's section. I suppose the "country club" side of Narco didn't apply to them. Horrified, Marie dreamed up schemes to get them outdoors, including drafting blueprints for the conversion of an abandoned yard into an outdoor recreation area. While she was awaiting permission for the project, she began to take the women on Sunday strolls around the grounds. One afternoon, a couple of the women used the opportunity to send notes to a few of the male patients, and staff found out. As this was strictly against the rules, the walks came to an end. Soon thereafter, one of the female patients destroyed all Marie's blueprints in a fit of rage. One of the older doctors chided her, "Marie, when you diagnose a patient as a psychopath, it figures she'll behave like one."

Reflecting on his words, Marie told the writer Nat Hentoff, "It was a good lesson for me. I had thought that in their respect for me and in their reaction to my great desire to help them, they'd all act differently. I had to learn that patients' own needs and particular sicknesses determine what they do. You can't function well with addicts, for example, if you try to gratify you own needs through them. They have more pressing problems than satisfying you."[59] If your motivations to "help" others were only based in a desire to feel better about yourself, you should probably reconsider.

Marie said that the women were "especially difficult. . . . Once, a big, tough girl dragged me into a room, insisting I give her the key to the drug cabinet. I didn't have it, so she roughed me up a little. It was frightening at times." I can imagine Marie chuckling here, using humor to lighten the memory as she often did.

She continued: "Occasionally they would riot, and the guards would ask me to go over there and reason with them." During one such instance, the women were setting fire to the curtains and mattresses. Marie walked into the middle of the chaos, fear pulsing through her veins, and offered them cigarettes as a peace offering. After talking for a bit, a semblance of calm seeped into the room.

"I can't tell you how I did it. Perhaps they were able to feel there was something in me, too, which resisted being in a prison. I was always breaking rules there without knowing it."

And sometimes she did know it—she just didn't care. Around Christmas, loneliness and sadness weighed heavily upon her patients. To create some holiday cheer, Marie decided to give out some morphine.[60] I imagine a twenty-six-year-old Marie drawing up syringes of morphine as the men lined up, an excited electricity buzzing through the air: Marie thrilled at the prospect of getting caught, the men unbelieving of their good fortune. Marie stooped next to the chair where her first patient sat and drove a needle into the flesh of his arm. The man would soon be replaced by another, and another.

When Dr. Isbell arrived in the expansive ward's doorway, it took him several seconds to register the scene in front of him. "Dr. Nyswander," he bellowed, "what exactly do you think you are doing?" His jaw hung open in shock, and his ruddy cheeks grew even redder with anger. He marched over to her, hands clenched into fists as he watched her laughing with the patients.

Perhaps Marie put her hand on his shoulder, trying to displace some of the tension. "It's much better than alcohol! And it's Christmas time—the boys need a little cheering up."

She winked at the patient sitting in the chair, his sleeve already rolled up. Although a supportive hoot sounded from somewhere in the crowd, Dr. Isbell quickly put an end to the whole thing. I'm surprised Marie was not fired.

Marie told Courtwright that the year at Narco was the hardest year of her life. "Prison is a terrible thing—if you have any kind of personality that cares about your fellow man, working at a prison will simply blow you up with rage and frustration."

At one point, she even thought of leaving and asking for a transfer to another post, but her commanding officer warned that leaving her first job prematurely wouldn't look good on her resume. His advice being reasonable, she decided to stick it out for the rest of the year. But, of course, that didn't mean it was any easier, and, to cope, she played piano in the chapel and punched a boxing bag in the gym until her "knuckles were black and blue."[61]

Luckily, the patients started to look out for her. One night while crying in bed, Marie heard a tapping outside her bedroom window.[62] Surprised, she wiped her tears and moved to the ledge, where she saw two patients who worked in the kitchen standing outside. They slid a milkshake and a sandwich onto the sill before waving goodbye. Soon, their delivery became a nightly occurrence. Other patients played jazz for her, something they usually only did for themselves, and made sure she was invited to all the best sessions.[63] When Baby Lawrence, a famous tap dancer, was about to perform in the laundry room, somebody always ran to get Marie.[64]

When her yearlong post finally came to an end, I picture Marie grabbing her already-packed-bags and leaving the grounds as soon as possible, excited to return to bustling New York City. She told Hentoff, "I never wanted to see another addict" after Narco. Within months, she would begin her psychiatry residency at Bellevue Psychiatric Hospital and coursework in Freudian psychoanalysis at New York Medical College, trying everything she could to leave her foray into addiction medicine far behind.

CHAPTER 5

Flight

2019

Now that we had a newborn, city life was increasingly difficult. The grocery's parking lot was always full, and Finley's shrieks grew more incessant with each circle of the asphalt maze. When I finally found a spot, the adjoining car was usually so close that I didn't have enough space to swing the car seat out from the back. On the drive home, Finley's wails made the stop-and-go traffic even more intolerable. I wished I could soothe her, but pulling over, nursing, and then merging back on the freeway would tack an additional half-hour onto what should have been a fast excursion.

When I returned to work in the Alameda ED, Finley's transition to daycare did not go particularly well. On her first day, she cried incessantly and refused to take a bottle. After four hours, the daycare called me to pick her up. I assumed she would adapt, but, as the days passed, nothing changed. One afternoon, the daycare attendant told me that she left Finley in her car seat for the entire, eight-hour day, as she didn't cry quite as loudly when strapped in. When I asked why they hadn't tried holding her, they told me they didn't have enough staff—she and her husband watched ten kids who ranged in age from babies to seven-year-olds. Although I wished I could put Finley somewhere else, all the quality programs had waitlists hovering around two years.

During shifts, I struggled to find the time and space to pump. Our ED was so small that only one doctor worked at a time, so even taking fifteen minutes to pump meant that I was often late to traumas or cardiac arrests. When I tried the "discreet" pump that fit into my bra so I could pump even while seeing patients, I developed painful, clogged ducts that later required hours of care to resolve. Just as Marie didn't have the vision to see how a naval ship might accommodate women, I didn't know how a single-coverage ED could accommodate me, a breastfeeding physician, and I was too ashamed to ask, just as I had been too ashamed to speak up when they told me I wasn't eligible for paid maternity leave. Now I know that standing up for myself has the potential to help the women who come after me, but at the time, I didn't want them to see me as the problem I felt like I was. After Marie climbed beyond the glass ceiling, did she expect the women who followed to suck it up and face the same brutalities? Or did she try to make things better? Maybe she never broke through at all—despite all of her successes, she was seen by many as no more than the wife of the mastermind behind methadone maintenance.

Additionally, my work environment was increasingly hostile. The physician group that had staffed the ED for the last twenty years had been replaced by the one that I now worked for, and, as the new ED medical director and chair, I represented the face of change. It didn't help that I was a young woman. The medicine chair, a man several decades my senior, prohibited me from something as simple as speaking during meetings, which made it very difficult to do my job. When we worked together clinically, he would inevitably open his eyes wide, stutter admonishments, and then loudly criticize my medical care as "not how we do things here" before racing out of the ED or hanging up the phone. When one of the executive administrators argued with me about my title, insisting there was no way I could be chair, I wasn't sure how to respond. I was struggling, and what for? Just so my baby could cry for eight hours in a daycare she hated? So I could clock into a job that fought me every second of every day? I constantly felt like I was failing at both motherhood and my career, each one constantly demanding more of the other.

At home, Warren and I started to bicker more about stupid things, and it was getting harder to come up for air as the accrual of tedious days and nights pushed us further under water. One evening, we thought that going out to one of our favorite bars might help remind us of what it felt like to have fun, so we brought the baby and met friends at the open-air patio, a dog lounging in the corner. As I filled up a bowl with crispy popcorn so fresh that its hot butter burned the tip of my tongue, the bartender saw us and asked us to leave. No babies allowed. Our old life had kicked us out and slammed the door behind us.

Things at the startup weren't so great, either. Although the attorney had knocked the medical board complaint down to a fine, the investigation's reverberations lingered. In the early summer, I met with one of the CEOs for tea at a small cafe in the valley between Oakland and Berkeley. She had flown in from Michigan to woo more funding from venture capitalists, and now she was sitting in front of me with an ultimatum. She insisted it wasn't her doing—their board was making her do it—but there she was, straight-lipped and stern, nonetheless. If I refused to obtain a medical license in every state in which they operated, which they hoped would eventually be all fifty, they would have no other choice but to let me go. She told me they already had my replacement picked out, an eager ED-doc-turned-VC who knew nothing about addiction but was interested in startups. My chest caved in. That's who they thought would take the company to the next level? Couldn't they at least find someone with significant addiction medicine experience?

As I sipped my chai, I realized the time had come. The startup didn't pay enough to support our family or repay my loans, nor did it provide health insurance or retirement. And now it was also asking me to take risks that had already threatened my medical license and career as an emergency physician. It was just too much.

As I walked out of the cafe, a copper bell clanged against the door and reverberated with the disappointment tumbling out of my heart. I thought that working with women might be different, that being part of a disruptive team espousing idealist principles meant we would change the system for the better, but, in the end, it was still just business. Now what? Was I just going to return to being a regular ED doc? I kicked a pebble across the sidewalk and watched it tumble over the curb. Was that it for my career in addiction medicine? I felt the tug of loss from something I didn't even realize I wanted.

When Warren, Finley, and I stepped out of the Tucson airport, it was shockingly quiet. Where was the honking and shouting we had left behind? I squinted as we walked into the bright sun and past a tall green saguaro reaching its arms toward the blue sky. The air smelled like the earth—metal mixed with dust. Finley smiled and moved her palm in the air, grasping for something still unseen.

I felt a pleasant nostalgia as we drove under rows of puffy white clouds stretching far into the distance, remembering the joyful years I spent earning my bachelor's at the University of Arizona. There is a Jewish adage, "Change your place, change your luck," and I thought that moving back to the wide-open skies of the desert might be exactly what I needed to bring a little more spaciousness to a life that was feeling increasingly stuck. A few months prior, I reached out to an acquaintance of mine who worked as a doc at the university. Although he told me they were not hiring, he suggested that I meet with their chair of emergency medicine so that when a job did open up, he might remember me. So here we were, feigning that we were in Tucson to visit friends when, really, we were just here for an unofficial interview scheduled the following day.

The medical school and university hospital occupied several blocks on the northern end of campus, their sleek modern architecture a stunning contrast against the classic brick of the historic buildings. The chair's office was spacious and surrounded by glass. He smiled as his assistant ushered me in to a scooped leather seat across from his desk, and I sat with my hands clasped in my lap. He was lean and tall, with short gray curls topping his head. Within the first five minutes of our conversation, he leaned forward and offered me a job. He hoped I could start as soon as possible.

When I got back to the rental car, I immediately called Warren. "Well, how did it go?" he asked.

"He offered me a job!" My heart pounded with excitement; I wanted to run and jump and dance. I looked toward the expansive horizon, toward our future.

"What? Really! I thought they didn't have any open positions?" He barely took a breath.

"That's what I thought, too! He said that in addition to working ED shifts, I would get to work with the residents and some fire departments in Southern Arizona. They will also support my research interests."

"That's exactly what you wanted!"

"Yeah, it sounds pretty great." Maybe an academic job would provide the satisfaction I had been unable to find as an ED medical director and had lost when leaving the startup.

"Well, what did you say?"

"I said I needed to think about it."

"Are you kidding? Why?"

"Well, we hadn't really talked about this as an option." I tapped my fingers on the gray dash. "And they don't have any opportunities for me to keep working in addiction." I frowned. Although I loathed my job at Alameda, stepping down after just a year felt like a personal failure, further evidence women shouldn't be ED directors or chairs. Because there had not been one big, dramatic event that pushed me out of this role, only a thousand tiny papercuts that worsened after the baby was born, it seemed silly to leave. But, according to researcher Renate Ysseldyk, my experience was not unique; this was the exact pattern that preceded the departure of so many women from academics.[1] Isabel Torres, the cofounder and chief executive of Mothers in Science, further explained that because the obstacles facing mothers in STEM are largely invisible, women, as well as those around them, assume that all it takes to succeed is hard work and determination. So when a woman finally chooses to walk away from the fallout of systemic failings, it is framed as a personal decision.[2] And that's exactly how I felt. Even though I wasn't leaving medicine or academics, I was making the opposite of a vertical career move, leaving a more prestigious, male-dominated role in leadership for an assistant professor position that paid significantly less.

Warren asked, "Did he ask about the medical board ruling?"

"No, but I don't think he knows."

"Are you going to tell him?"

"If I take the job, I will have to—credentialing applications always ask about that kind of thing." As would the Arizona Medical Board, which would delay my licensing by so many weeks that I almost had to push back my start date and reschedule my first shifts—not the best first impression.

"Anyway," Warren continued, "the position sounds great, you hate your job in California, and we love Tucson. Maybe you can find a way to include addiction later."

I nodded. Without the added demands of urban life, maybe I'd even have time to start hiking again, baby in tow. Untamped joy started to build in my chest. At last, we had found a way home.

At first, I was good about saying no to extra opportunities at work. In the mornings, I'd buckle Finley, now almost one-year-old, into her carrier, swing the heavy contraption around my hip, and slide my arms through its straps before trekking through the dramatic rock formations of the Tucson Mountains or the narrow, climbing canyons of the Santa Catalinas. I loved hearing the chattering of the cactus wren and spotting their nests magnificently coiled around the sharp spikes of cholla. Once, we found ourselves in the middle of a summer monsoon, just like the one that had ambushed Marie and her friend decades ago. The air smelled like creosote, earthy and sweet, and my soaked clothes felt refreshingly cool against the afternoon heat. Finley smiled toward the heavens, exuberant. But only a month passed before I couldn't hold myself back anymore.

It started innocently enough. Carl, the university hospital's EMS coordinator, was taking me to meet the fire chiefs of Santa Cruz County, a sparsely populated, rolling country that stretched between Tucson and Sonora, Mexico. There were a handful of fire departments in the county, miles and miles between each one, and I was their new medical director. Any time someone called 911 for medical assistance, their EMTs and paramedics responded. Carl wanted to make sure the chiefs had a face to go with the name, as handshakes went a long way in Fire. We started with Nogales, a city split in two by the tall metal bars of the US-Mexico border.

A firefighter dressed in a black uniform met us at the station's front door and ushered us into an office. There sat the chief, a man with black hair wearing a white button-down shirt tucked into pressed slacks. He stood and extended his hand, his large, wide palm encircling mine. As we settled into our leather chairs, he launched into his goals for improving the department's medical care, the conversation quickly drifting to opioids. "Fentanyl is a real problem around here," the chief explained. "Lately, it seems to be everywhere." He leaned forward at his desk, his weight resting on his hefty forearms.

Fifty times stronger than heroin, fentanyl is a synthetic opioid manufactured in illicit labs. Some users prefer the more intense high provided by fentanyl, purposely purchasing the blue pills known around here as "Mexican Blues" or "M30s." Others just can't find any heroin or pills without fentanyl, as it is so much cheaper to manufacture. Some of my patients tell me they can buy a tablet for as little as a dollar. Because it is man-made, there is no need to worry about weather conditions; there will always be a good harvest. Because it is highly concentrated, small quantities worth a lot of money can easily be hidden and smuggled. All of that is to say it seems impossible to curtail its supply.

Fentanyl's extreme potency also makes it more likely to cause a fatal overdose by respiratory depression. Because its production is not regulated, there are over twenty analogues that street fentanyl can contain, each with slightly different strengths and properties, and nobody knows exactly what they are getting. Whereas we had thought oxycodone was a big problem back in the early 2000s, now it seemed relatively mild when compared to the skyrocketing number of overdoses attributable to fentanyl.

The chief continued: "At my last job in Washington State, we had a robust leave-behind naloxone program, and I'd love to start something like that here."

My ears piqued with interest. "Oh, really?"

Naloxone is an opioid antagonist, meaning it kicks heroin and fentanyl off the brain's opioid receptors. If spritzed up the nose of someone who had just overdosed, their chest would heave with breath, color would return to their lips, and their eyes would slowly flicker open. And if it were accidentally given to someone who didn't have opioids in their system, nothing would happen. No harm, no foul.

Yet, despite naloxone's ease and safety, it was relatively hard to get. Back then, it was not sold over the counter, so users had to first visit a doctor and get a prescription. Additionally, some pharmaceutical companies charged exorbitant amounts for their unique medication delivery systems. And although most first responders carried naloxone, they didn't always get there in time, especially in rural counties. Additionally, some people were too scared to call 911 when their friends overdosed, worried that any cops who arrived might arrest them.

To overcome such obstacles, activists developed programs to get naloxone into the hands of the people who needed it most—users like them—by giving it out for free and without a prescription. As users were the ones who best understood the problem, they, not the doctors, were the ones who came up with the solution. For decades, naloxone's use had been limited to an ivory tower of hospitals and ambulances, far out of reach from the people who needed it most. Overdose was seen as an inevitable consequence of heroin use. But, in the 1990s, a handful of activists across the country found a way to get naloxone, teach others how to use it, and distribute it among their friends, even though doing so meant they risked arrest and jail time. Here in Arizona, Haley Coles grew such a grassroots program into one of the biggest naloxone distributors in the country, Sonoran Prevention Works. Now, such naloxone leave-behind programs are a staple component of our country's public health response—but it wasn't always like that.

Although studies overwhelmingly confirmed that this simple intervention reduces overdose fatalities, opponents still believed that naloxone distribution was enabling; if people knew that an overdose was less likely to kill them, maybe they would feel a little too comfortable getting high.[3] But that wasn't how addiction worked, a defining characteristic of substance use disorder being the continued use despite the harm. Additionally, study after study showed that naloxone programs actually led to decreased use.[4] When people felt that their lives mattered, they slowly started to make safer choices. But, regardless, didn't users deserve to live whether or not they continued to use? Wasn't preventing death the primary goal?

Although layperson naloxone programs were supported by the likes of the World Health Organization, the American Medical Association, the American Public Health Association, and the National Association of Boards of Pharmacy, many EMS agencies still considered them to be experimental and outside of their scope. Although modern EMS had developed in the 1960s to respond to the major cause of accidental death at the time—modern vehicle accidents—most agencies hadn't appropriately pivoted to treat today's leading cause of accidental death: overdose. Like the rest of medicine, they thought treating addiction was best left to someone else.

"I would love to start a program like that," I answered.

"Great, Gerry here will help you," said the chief, patting the shoulder of a man who had just walked in.

Gerry's dark black hair was gelled to the side, and a corner of his lip curved upward in a half-smile. "Yeah, sure, we can do that," he said. "Just let me know what you need, Doc."

But Gerry didn't wait. Only a few days passed before he nudged me. "Just send us the protocols and the training, and we can get it going."

When a few weeks passed and I still hadn't sent the documents, he emailed that several of our fire departments would be attending an opioid consortium meeting in Nogales, and they'd like me to present on our leave-behind program. I promised I'd be there, protocols in hand.

The meeting was held in a brick building about one hundred yards from the US-Mexico border, with representatives from the school, police, border patrol, peer recovery, fire department, and local clinic all in attendance. Breakfast was set out buffet-style on the large folded table, and chairs were arranged in a square around the room. Once the session began, an epidemiologist with long curly hair stood to present her data, passing out stapled packets as she spoke. According to her research, chaotic opioid use was much more common on the US side.

When it was time for questions, a man with a scruffy auburn beard and scowling eyebrows shot his hand in the air. His eyes darted from the printed papers in his hands, up to the speaker, and back down again as he began: "In your needs assessment, you state that users often have a history of trauma. But you didn't mention that incarceration is a source of trauma. Incarcerating people for drug use is traumatic." He kept his eyes focused on hers, waiting for a response.

I shuffled uncomfortably in my seat. I mean, yes, he was right, but, come on, nobody in this room could change that. His accusations seemed unnecessarily confrontational, like he was blaming this poor epidemiologist for the entire drug war. How would the audience react? Although nobody in the room had an answer, peoples' faces remained kind, and a few even nodded. Then somebody else raised their hand, carrying the conversation off in a different direction.

The man went back to reading the packet, seemingly ignoring the discussion. He was wearing dark jeans and a leather jacket, not the uniform of police or healthcare worker, a clue that perhaps he was the man Haley Coles recommended I meet here today. Christopher Thomas was the Sonoran Prevention Works overdose prevention coordinator assigned to Santa Cruz County, and I hoped he would be willing to supply our fire departments with free naloxone kits. Because Sonoran Prevention Works was part of a harm reduction buyers' club similar to those born during the 1980s AIDS epidemic, they were able to buy naloxone for only a dollar a dose, something our fire departments couldn't do.[5] As some of our fire departments were so small that they were mainly staffed by volunteers, free was our only option.

But there was no time to discreetly introduce myself; as soon as the epidemiologist sat down, it was time for me to present about our proposed leave-behind naloxone project. Anytime our firefighters reversed someone's overdose, they would also give a naloxone kit to that person or their friends and family. When I clicked to the slide outlining the content that I wanted to include in the firefighters' training, I looked to Christopher as I suggested, "Maybe we can work together to make sure the content is robust enough." He raised his eyebrows and nodded. *Good.*

The next slide highlighted Arizona's Good Samaritan law. I explained, "According to Arizona Revised Statute 13–3421, if somebody calls 911 for a drug related overdose, neither the person calling nor the person overdosing can be charged for possession."

Christopher's hand once again shot up. "But they still might get arrested," he said dryly as he looked over at the police officer in the room.

The officer shrugged her shoulders and calmly responded, "Well, although we won't arrest anyone for possession, we are still going to run everyone's record. That's just what we do when we arrive on scene. And if they have a warrant, we will take them in for that."

My eyebrows raised at the sinister implication of this approach. It didn't seem far-fetched that people with chaotic drug use or financial insecurity might collect a few warrants along the way, even just an unpaid ticket for sleeping outside. If law enforcement continued to arrest people, what use was a Good Samaritan law? I would later learn that this was a common issue across the country, with such laws failing to adequately protect those who called for help.[6]

After the meeting ended, Christopher stood and packed his papers into his bag, not bothering to make small talk with anyone. I maneuvered my way through the crowd, waving at the various medics I recognized, before reaching him. "Christopher?" I asked, extending a hand.

He looked up, a smile landing on his face. "You must be Melody."

"Yes, I'm glad we could meet here today."

"Your program sounds good."

"Oh, great." Relief relaxed the muscles in my face. "Do you have any train the trainer sessions coming up that I could attend? So I could get a better of idea of best practices for teaching the medics how to train bystanders?"

Again, he nodded. "Yes, we do. I'll send you the invite."

Back in Tucson, a volunteer with purple hair greeted me as I stepped through the front door of the Southern Arizona AIDS Foundation, the corner storefront of a mainly abandoned office park. Taking my seat in the large meeting room, I noticed that the harm reduction crowd was a lot hipper than the doctors and firefighters I usually worked with. One woman in particular caught my eye, as something about her felt familiar. She had wavy dark hair cut in the long layers of a shag, capped by a red beanie. On her face she wore gold, wire-rimmed aviator glasses, and on her legs tight black jeans that rode high over leather Blundstones. Dark, unshaven hair sprouted from her shins. She reminded me of the punks that I used to hang out with at the bicycle cooperative in college, the ones who sometimes hopped the freight trains. It felt both exciting and comforting to have found my way back to this bohemian scene, a little like Marie among her jazz musicians.

Harm reduction was a philosophy often mentioned in addiction medicine, although its tenets could be applied to almost any aspect of healthcare. Harm reduction was fastening your seatbelt when you got into a car, slathering on sunblock when you lay on the beach, injecting insulin when you indulged in a slice of cake. As a term, it was first coined in 1987 to describe both a philosophy and a practice aimed at reducing the dangers associated with illicit drug use.[7] Key to harm reduction is the grassroots doctrine "Nothing about us without us," elevating the priorities of people who use drugs above those of physicians or elected officials. It is also rooted in realism; not everyone is ready to quit using drugs, so why not help them do so more safely? People with a substance use disorder will find ways to use, whether or not they have a clean needle—that is the defining diagnostic criteria of addiction. So, let's help them stay alive until, or if, they are ready to stop using.

Because harm reduction supports any positive change, abstinence is not always the end goal. That might not always look pretty, as many people with chaotic drug use do get sick, lose their families, become homeless. Harm reduction does not deny this. Instead, self-determination and body autonomy are the targets, treating users as the experts in their own lives. On the ground, harm reduction looks like giving out naloxone, fentanyl test strips, and clean syringes and pipes. In some places, it even means drug decriminalization, overdose prevention sites, and a safe supply. It means that we don't push buprenorphine or methadone on people. We support any positive change.

Although I agreed with this in theory, in practice part of me wasn't so sure. Many addiction doctors downplayed the importance of harm reduction, instead insisting that treatment with buprenorphine, and maybe methadone, was the real way forward. At the time, I agreed with them. Of course, I still thought it was a good idea to hand out naloxone; I was here, wasn't I? But I wasn't so sure how I felt about passing out clean pipes, or even syringes. How did handing out pipes help people? If Sonoran Prevention Works gave out too many syringes, would we start to see them littered upon the ground?

Later, I would read studies showing that such programs actually decrease the number of improperly-disposed-of needles,[8] as well as rates of drug use,[9] crime,[10] needle stick injuries,[11] and the spread of infectious diseases.[12] But, perhaps equally important, giving out pipes and syringes is a way to build trust with people who use drugs; when they say that is what they need to stay safer, we listen.

Unfortunately, it was illegal. Until the summer of 2021, passing out pipes and syringes was a felony under Arizona state paraphernalia laws. When Haley cofounded Sonoran Prevention Works in 2010, she was particularly worried about provoking the ire of Sheriff Joe Arpaio, who had promised to personally arrest anyone who provided clean syringes. This was no small threat. Sheriff Joe's tent city, an outdoor jail where inmates slept on metal bunk beds under green canopies left over from the Korean War, frequently appeared in the national news for its abuses of human rights. In the summer, temperatures could reach 130 degrees Fahrenheit, and in the winter, near freezing. As if that wasn't bad enough, Maricopa County also ran the last all-female chain gang in the country and bragged about it.[13] Despite the risk, Sonoran Prevention Works did it anyway.

Christopher stood at the front of the room, preparing his slides. After our first meeting in Nogales, he agreed to provide our fire departments with free naloxone. Today, I planned to ask if Sonoran

Prevention Works could also supply our emergency department so we could start a hospital-based program. Although I had tried not to go above and beyond at work, to just stick to my prescribed job duties, I could no longer hold myself back. The more I worked in Arizona, the more I stumbled upon gaps in addiction care. Setting up the leave-behind naloxone program with Nogales Fire swung open some door that I could no longer shut, reminding me that I could not leave addiction medicine behind.

I also realized that the emergency department was the perfect place for outreach. Because many patients with chaotic use lacked health insurance, a primary care provider, or even a working phone, they came to the ED when they needed help. We were the safety net. Yet few EDs started MOUD or gave out naloxone. If I didn't change that, it felt like nobody would. With those kinds of stakes, how could I walk away?

Soon, Christopher began his presentation, and, once again, I found his brusque tone off-putting. He complained about people who didn't use person-first language when talking about people with chaotic drug use, claiming they were the same people who didn't care about the humanity of people who use drugs. But, before today, I hadn't even heard of the term "person first" language. I shifted uncomfortably in my seat. What did that say about me?

But the more Christopher spoke, the more his words stuck. "People love my personal narrative," he began. "I was shooting up meth, went to prison, and then got clean. Now I dress nicely, I give lectures, and I am a father. Blah blah blah." He took some time to look at us. "But not everyone's plotline looks like that. At any one time, only about 5 percent of users want to stop their chaotic usage, so we need to meet them where they are. We need to use harm reduction. But let's take a step back. First, let's talk about stigma."[14]

He showed us a slide with an image of heroin next to an image of alcohol. "What is the difference between these two substances? Stigma, criminalization, and acceptable harm." He clicked to a photo of several glasses of beer and liquor and said "In 2015, the National Institutes of Health estimated that eighty-eight thousand people die every year from alcohol-related causes, making alcohol the third leading preventable cause of death in the US. In 2014, drunk driving accounted for over 30 percent of overall driving fatalities. Almost one hundred thousand college-age students were a victim of alcohol-related sexual assault or date rape. But what do we do about it? As a society, we have decided that the harms associated with alcohol are acceptable. The benefits outweigh the harms." Then he clicked to a slide showing heroin. "With heroin, we have stigmatized not only the drug itself, but its users, as well."

I found myself nodding in agreement.

As he panned through the slides about the philosophy of harm reduction, he continued: "Sometimes people tell me that distributing Narcan is sending the wrong message. I don't know what they mean when they say this. When we give someone naloxone, we are telling them that we care about them. That we love them. That they do not deserve to die from an overdose.

"Sometimes people ask me, 'How many times do I have to give Narcan to the same person?,' frustrated that they see the same person overdosing more than once. I tell them, 'If it were your sister, how many times would you want me to revive her? As many times as it takes!'"

I began to understand the weary frustration in his voice, but it wouldn't be until months later that I would feel it myself. I wondered how many times he had given this same presentation, how many more it would take to convince people to care. And why should he have to? Shouldn't it be obvious that everyone deserves to be treated with basic human decency? That, just because you used drugs, you didn't deserve to die? In the face of how many people were needlessly dying, perhaps it was okay to be a little appalled, to be a little angry. Anything less felt callous.

At the end of the session, Christopher held my gaze while making his closing comments to the room. "If you are in a position of power to make treatment and policy decisions, make sure we have those with a history of chaotic use at the table. And make sure they are compensated for their time."

CHAPTER 6

Roped Back

1947

In 1947, Marie began her psychiatry residency at Manhattan's Bellevue Psychiatric Hospital, a brick building that looked stately on a sunny day but imposing during the gray of winter.[1] As a resident, Marie still held on to notions of addiction that she had absorbed at Narco—namely, "that addicts were the lowest form of creature," and "they should all be sent to Lexington for treatment."[2] Relieved that her days of working in addiction were behind her, she dove into her psychoanalysis studies and dreamed about opening a private practice in Manhattan after residency.

One afternoon, Marie was jotting an order into a patient's thick blue binder at the nurse's station—or, at least, this is how I imagine this scene—when she heard the scream of a nurse down the hall: "She's seizing!"

Several other nurses were now running down the hallway, and one called out to her, "Doc, we need your help!"

Marie joined them as she jogged down the corridor, her pumps clacking against the linoleum. Peering into one of the rooms, her gaze narrowed on the patient in question. She was in her forties, her hair disheveled around her pointed face, and she was most definitely seizing.

Marie asked, "What's her history?"

"She has anxiety and depression," one of the nurses answered. "She checked in two days ago."

"No prior seizures?" Marie questioned.

The nurse shook her head.

"Is she on any medications?"

"She had been on pentobarbital, but the intern cut her off," the nurse answered.

"He did what?!" Barbiturates were a highly addictive class of medication, often used during Marie's day to treat anxiety and insomnia. When abruptly stopped, they caused seizures and even death. At Narco, she had learned how to detox patients dependent on barbiturates by gradually decreasing their dose. But this intern had no idea. In 1947, these medications were still believed to be so safe that a prescription wasn't required, and it wouldn't be until the 1950s that reliable evidence for barbiturate dependence was published.[3] Marie only knew better because of what she had seen at Narco.

Marie shouted, "Give her sodium amytal, stat!"[4]

The nurse ran to the cabinet, drew up the medication, and injected the clear solution into the woman's IV. And, just like that, the seizure was over, the patient now sleeping soundly.

Marie told Courtwright, "How can you walk away when there is a woman . . . starting to convulse? You cannot not treat that woman. And on it goes." Over the months and years that followed, Marie continued to find herself in situations where she felt compelled to act, soon becoming Bellevue's de facto addiction specialist. Any time a doctor had a question about dependence or addiction, it was Marie they consulted. If a patient arrived in withdrawal at midnight, they would call Marie. But this wasn't the career she wanted. To put an end to all this, one of her colleagues recommended that she write an article about withdrawal. Marie thought, "Oh, great, I'll write a paper and then I won't ever have to see another addict, and everybody will know how to do it."[5]

So, her first academic paper was published in 1950, and not just anywhere, but in the prestigious *New England Journal of Medicine*.[6] Quite a boon for a resident. But the resulting impact was not quite what she had hoped. As she told Courtwright, "Of course what that did was set me up as an authority and so, far from being rid of the problem, more calls." Soon, she was not only the addiction expert for Bellevue Psychiatric Hospital, but for all of New York City, a trend that, despite her best intentions, continued beyond residency.

After she graduated, her first psychiatry job was in a swanky Park Avenue office. Her patients were solidly middle and upper class—discontented businessmen and bored housewives—and none suffered from addiction, just like she wanted.[7] But physicians kept calling her for advice. Marie said, "At the time, I was one of the only three psychotherapists in New York who had been at Lexington. As people became more alarmed about the increase in addiction, we were more and more sought out in crises. The other two finally backed out of the whole problem. They wouldn't handle any addicts. I didn't throw up my hands, perhaps because I'm a woman and was therefore enough of a masochist to go on."[8]

I imagine her laughing here, as she usually did when a topic ventured too close to some emotional core.

"As a result of the paper and of other doctors' knowledge that I was treating addicts, I eventually became inundated with them. People would call me up and I'd assume the obligation, handling addicts in whatever stumbling way I could because there was hardly anyone else."[9] She added, "If the problem came up, you had to respond to it if you knew how to do something."

Decades later, when Marie was in her sixties and a famous addiction physician, Courtwright asked, "Did you ever feel that you were trapped into the field? Have you ever had any regrets? Have you ever thought that you should have focused your talents on some other aspect of psychiatry?"

She didn't even need a second to think about her response, "Well, to answer your first question, did I feel trapped, yes, I felt trapped, especially in the beginning." A tone of fatigue momentarily crept into her voice—"I felt trapped into the field"—before her characteristic momentum returned and propelled her forward. "I really was gung-ho in psychoanalysis and this darn drug addiction would come up all the time, and I had something nag away, answer the question, do something about it." She stuttered, "I, I think if there had just been one other person in this city that would see addicts, I would probably have washed my hands, but there wasn't anybody and you can't abandon them"—she laughed—"at least in the way I was raised, you simply can't abandon someone when there's nobody to give you a glass of water, you know," and her conclusion rushed out, "so, in a way, I was trapped."

My path into addiction medicine felt similarly happenstance, prompted by the shocking lack of alternatives for my patients. But I didn't resist quite as much as Marie had. Until addiction medicine found me, I was bumbling about in the dark. Now I finally had the purpose I had been looking for. Yet I could relate with the sense of claustrophobia. The work was never-ending, it didn't pay particularly well, and there weren't enough addiction physicians to share the load. But if I walked away, what would happen to my patients?

Marie then responded to Courtwright's second question, did she have any regrets, anything that she wished she had done differently? "No, nothing. I think it's just been one of the more fortunate things that ever happened. As a doctor you have to work with some group of patients, and I can't tell you what a rewarding group of patients they are—anybody who has worked with them will say the same thing—it isn't just me. It's just a very rewarding group of people and they're so brave; the magnitude of change as I said before is, there's just nothing like it." A door squeaked in the background, and Marie laughed. "And it requires very little work. I think I must be lazy because they mainly do it themselves. All you have to do is just be halfway decent and friendly and a joke now and then, try to remove some guilt from them and boy, they just go ahead. So, I would say that it's just a very fortunate thing. I will die with a smile on my face because of this accident of working with addicts."

1950s

When Marie first started fielding addiction questions from other physicians, she initially regurgitated lots of Narco dogma. "We had a little cliché treatment for them that we believed in," she explained.[10] But the more patients she helped, the more she met whose situation didn't fit the mold. Although physicians feel more comfortable in the black and white of textbooks, the reality is that most people and their illnesses live in the gray.

One morning, a physician from New Jersey called for advice about an elderly man who had become addicted to pain medications after surgery. Marie, only half listening because she was reading the review of a recent jazz album, blurted out her automatic response: "He needs to go Narco."[11]

Marie had been taught that withdrawals were too dangerous to manage at home and could only occur during a hospitalization. Now this notion seems silly. It also seemed like every patient would know better, having accidentally gone through withdrawals before when their supply ran low. But I guess doctors weren't in the habit of taking suggestions from their patients back then. Further supporting the perceived need for institutionalization was the prevalent stereotype that addicts were potentially dangerous, criminal, poorly motivated, and just plain untreatable.[12]

There was an audible hesitancy on the other end of the line. "But he's an old man. You can't send him to prison. He'll probably die there."

Hadn't Marie seen firsthand the horrors created by the carceral atmosphere of Lexington? She wouldn't want her own father sent there; why should she wish this on someone else's? "So, are you suggesting a home detox?" she asked.

"Yes, yes, I am."

Marie paused. "Don't you think that he will somehow still obtain drugs? That the man will probably convince his wife or kids to sneak him some pills?"

"No, I think he's pretty committed to this, and his family is supportive."

Marie nodded, excitement building for the challenge at hand. "Okay. Well, here is what I would recommend . . ." diving into a gradually decreasing, four-times-a-day morphine regimen. She could hear the physician furiously scribbling down her instructions on his notepad. Every day, he called her to check in. Within three weeks, the man had successfully withdrawn from opioids, proving to Marie that home detox *was* possible.[13] In the years that followed, she would supervised hundreds more.

However, Marie herself never actually prescribed any opioids for home withdrawals. She couldn't—she didn't have a narcotics license. As she told Hentoff, "My commanding officer at Lexington had advised me not to get a license, because once addicts knew I had one, they'd keep pressing me to give them drugs. But the real reason I didn't apply was that if a doctor prescribes narcotics for drug addicts, he runs the risk of having to defend his use of the license to the Federal Bureau of Narcotics, and I was a coward. I wasn't prepared emotionally or financially for court battles. Informers, incidentally, had been sent to my office from time to time to see if I ever referred patients to doctors who would give them drugs. I never did."[14] Harry Anslinger, the head of the DEA's predecessor and the architect of America's war on drugs, had made it quite clear that he would go after any doctor who so much as gave a shot of morphine to an addict.[15]

Once again, Marie and I were fighting the same battles more than fifty years apart: the risk of medical board investigations, the national debate over demand versus supply, healthcare versus incarceration. Marie's decision to forego a narcotics license turned out to be the right choice; if she had lost her medical license, she wouldn't have been able to work with Vince at Rockefeller, and methadone maintenance may never have been invented. But how did one decide how much risk was too much?

Over my office desk, I had taped an Audre Lorde quote to the wall: "The master's tools will never dismantle the master's house." Time and time again, it was radical grassroots movements that had brought healthcare and justice to vulnerable communities, not the so-called "leaders." During the AIDS epidemic of the 1980s, it was queer men with AIDS illicitly distributing antiretrovirals to their friends, as the alternative, waiting for the FDA to approve this new treatment, was equivalent to a death sentence. In the 1990s, it was drug users who democratized naloxone by developing leave-behind programs.[16] But how did this model apply to someone like me, someone working within the system?

I suspected that the path forward could be found in allyship, which, at its core, I believe requires some amount of risk, a spectrum ranging from risking political capital by voicing an unpopular opinion to risking arrest by disobeying unjust laws. But where to draw the line?

Reading the notes from a 1993 interview between historian David Courtwright and Charles Winick, it seemed like Marie also mulled over this balance between making change from outside the system versus from within. She even considered prescribing opioids precisely so she could get arrested and serve as a test case. After all, when she was a teenage activist, she was not afraid to break the law. But now she had more to lose. If she were arrested, she would be treated as a pariah by her colleagues and wouldn't be allowed to practice medicine until the trial's resolution, effectively abandoning her patients. So she decided to keep toeing the line. At least somewhat.

In 1955, Marie and Charles Winick, a sociologist whom she met while volunteering on the board of directors for Narcotics Anonymous, created a voluntary outpatient treatment program called the Narcotic Addiction Research Project.[17] Under their model, a patient could participate in psychoanalysis and group therapy during the day and still make it home in time for dinner, an impossible scenario anywhere else in New York because the medical community still believed that addicts needed to be institutionalized. Furthermore, abstinence would not be a precondition for treatment—another radical notion back then. As Marie asked, "How can you ask them to get off drugs when that's their problem?"[18]

Marie financed the whole operation herself, hiring a secretary, seven psychiatrists, eleven psychologists, and twelve social workers. And, although they did not have a physical clinic in which to meet, somehow they made it work.[19] Even though "harm reduction" was not yet a term, their team already practiced its patient-centered tenets. Marie wrote, "The patients' own motivations were accepted, and the staff was willing to work with them at whatever level they were willing to work." She met them where they were. Additionally, she wrote that their "therapeutic goal was the treatment of the total individual rather than his drug addiction."[20] Even today, many physicians are not so progressive.

Marie and Winick's results were published in 1957, proving that patients with addiction could be treated on an outpatient basis alongside other medical patients instead of being shipped off to Narco.[21] Although outpatient treatment is now mainstream, the underlying argument for increased access is still relevant; instead of isolating patients to methadone clinics—a service not even available in about half of the country—wouldn't it be nice if they could get a methadone prescription from their primary care clinic, a practice currently prohibited by federal regulation? Wouldn't it be nice if physicians from all specialties offered buprenorphine instead of the measly 2 percent who prescribe it now? But, in the 1950s, Marie's approach wasn't just controversial; it was revolutionary, and it wasn't long before she was identified as a heretic who needed to be silenced.

When the Federal Bureau of Narcotics caught wind of what Marie and Winick were up to, they sent an agent, Samuel Levine, to attend every one of their staff meetings.[22] For once, Marie was glad she didn't have a narcotics license, as it would have been the perfect excuse for Levine to arrest her. It seemed like he was always trying to find some way to turn her into a cautionary tale to deter other doctors from treating addiction. Marie told Courtwright that she found an official report confirming the bureau's systematic intimidation of anyone and everyone working in outpatient addiction, part of a strategy to scare doctors into just giving up.[23] For the most part, it seemed to work.

Marie felt so targeted that she hired a lawyer to help, but once he heard what she was doing, he panicked. I could just imagine his eyebrows lifting, wrinkles stretching from temple to temple, his speech becoming pressured, beads of sweat forming on his upper lip as he tried to convince Marie to just drop her project, to forget about it, waving his hands around or nervously shuffling papers. When she told Courtwright about her attorney's concerns, she playfully minimized the situation, "He went through all this mish mosh—he was very concerned." Although this jaunty tone might fool most listeners, I knew how stressful it was to be the target of a medical investigation.

Additionally, Anslinger did not mess around. Just a few years prior, he had successfully pushed Congress to pass the Boggs Act, setting mandatory sentences for drug convictions. If someone were arrested for marijuana possession, they faced a minimum sentence of two to ten years. Anslinger had gained support for the act by successfully stoking the flames of white America's racial fears, linking marijuana to crazed Mexicans and Black men sleeping with white women.[24] When the American Medical Association (AMA) published a report debunking many of Anslinger's claims, he threatened to fire any of his agents who read it. When a professor argued that addicts needed compassionate care, not incarceration, Anslinger had him wiretapped and falsely told his university that he was involved with a "criminal organization."[25] If Marie made any misstep, Anslinger wouldn't have thought twice about making her life a living hell.

In Courtwright's interview with Marie, he asked, "Did you ever meet Anslinger?"

Marie answered with a deep laugh, "Oh, my, yes, I should say so."

Courtwright asked, "What was he like?"

Marie responded, "Well, I wouldn't say I knew him personally. He walked out every time I would be someplace. I can only tell you what his appearance was. His appearance was like a movie character of a death squad." She paused before continuing. "That's not very fair. . . . He was kind of baldish, a very thick neck, a very ruddy complexion, and didn't smile much, at least not to me he didn't, and was very critical. . . He was a very powerful man, perhaps the most powerful man in Washington."

In the late 1950s, Marie was invited to present her research at the National Research Council.[26] I pictured her standing behind a dark wood podium elevated on a small stage, wearing a shin-length dress and pearls, lecturing to an audience of mostly white male physicians. As she explained how she had provided outpatient psychoanalysis to patients who were still using, she couldn't help but notice the looks of scorn and incredulity upon the faces of her colleagues. Then, to top it off, she watched as Anslinger stood up, crimson anger stretching across his face. The men sitting around him, also in dark suits, followed his lead, and, together, they all marched out, down the center aisle, sending an unspoken message to the rest of the crowd. One of his agents later said, "Anybody that came out with any academic work that could be critical of him, his Bureau, or his philosophy, had to go to prison, or be beheaded."[27]

After her presentation, Marie was chatting with a few other scientists and physicians near the stage when a biochemist came to shake her hand. He looked pleasant enough, smiling as he approached nearer. "Dr. Nyswander," he started, both his hands now wrapped around hers, "I must tell you, we felt that we shouldn't even invite you here because this is so immoral, what you're doing."[28]

Whereas I would have been shocked by such a statement, Marie took it in stride, chuckling to lighten the tension. Later, she would even describe him as a lovely man. I don't know if I would have been so generous. Then up came the executive secretary of the National Research Council's Committee on Drug Addiction, who made no pretense of being polite. He flat out told her that she ought to have her license removed.

Later, Marie would insist, perhaps a little too much, that there was absolutely no component of gender discrimination behind their chagrin, but, based on my own experiences, I had to wonder: As a woman, did they think she would be more easily intimidated? Did they think her ideas more foolish?

Although Marie had commented that this era was difficult for addicts, I imagine it was also difficult for her. She and a handful of her colleagues were the only ones who seemed to care about those who suffered from addiction, and the approach they advocated was dismissed as a screwball idea. Did she ever doubt her vision? According to a statement she made to Courtwright, I believe she did: "When you find yourself doing something nobody else does, it behooves you to ask, 'Am I out of line?'"

How did she find the emotional energy to keep pushing ahead in the face of so much criticism? Especially when the majority of her patients still relapsed? What was this time like for Marie, this time before she was famous, before the dramatic success of methadone maintenance was realized, before buprenorphine, before the formation of addiction medicine as a specialty complete with its own prestigious fellowship training programs? In this time, when her colleagues thought she was an eccentric crackpot? It must have been exceedingly lonely. Perhaps I knew a little how that felt.

———

For months, I had been trying to convince our hospital administration to approve my emergency department naloxone program. Studies showed that less than 2 percent of naloxone prescriptions were filled by patients after leaving the ED, so I wanted to place a package of naloxone directly into the palm of their hand. Sonoran Prevention Works and the local health department both agreed to give us free naloxone, no strings attached, so our hospital would not have to spend a dime. I knew that asking the hospital to spend money on patients with chaotic drug use—a population that didn't generate a lot of profit—would be too much. However, I didn't expect that it would be so hard just to give out free naloxone.

The first person at the hospital whom I approached with the idea was the medical director of our emergency department, Dr. Melissa Zukowski. She was the first female medical director I'd ever worked for, and, so far, the experience had been fantastic. When one of the residents and I needed a room to pump, she cleared out a nearby room, hung decorations on the wall, and bought a mini-fridge to store the milk. She, too, was a mom and hated that nurses and doctors had been pumping in the ED bathrooms, a place where the film of dried urine stuck to your shoe. I promised Melissa that this program would not take even a minute of her time—I was happy to do all the legwork. Without even missing a beat, Melissa agreed to help, suggesting that we first approach hospital pharmacy.

That's where the support ran dry. The head of pharmacy quickly dismissed the idea, simply proclaiming it as a policy violation. When I asked more questions, she said it would be too difficult for me to understand. I was confused by her opposition. The naloxone was free. It saved lives. Research even suggested that such programs saved money for hospitals. I sent her studies and citations in case she didn't believe me. None of it worked.

The program's rollout ground to a stop. Months went by. If I woke at three in the morning, my mind always turned to naloxone, and it was impossible to fall back asleep. During those dark, quiet hours before sunrise, I brainstormed new tactics to break this stalemate. At one point, I even asked Melissa if she would be mad if a box of naloxone just "appeared" in the emergency department, unclear who brought it there. She smiled, as if I were joking.

When I vented to an addiction physician in California about all the obstacles I kept facing when trying to expand our hospital's addiction services, she asked me, "Are you doing this all alone?"

I looked into her eyes, tears welling in my own. At the time, I was, and, once again, I wished I had someone to guide me through.

Despite the intimidation Marie faced from the Bureau of Narcotics, she felt encouraged by the results of her and Winick's Narcotic Addiction Research Project. If addiction treatment could be offered on an outpatient basis, it could be expanded more easily across the city and brought directly into the communities who needed it most. In 1957, she and Winick created a clinic for jazz musicians with addiction, and, in 1958, Dr. Beatrice Bishop Berle invited her to join her family medicine practice in East Harlem.

The clinic was located on East 100th Street between First and Second Avenues, an area that *The New York Times Magazine* called the city's "worst block." Dr. Berle described the buildings as being five-to-six story walk-ups with a "bathtub in the kitchen, a toilet in the hall, and uncertain lighting and heating." They also had a bit of a rat infestation, the rodents' "little beady eyes peering up through the holes in the floor."[29]

Initially, the clinic did not offer addiction treatment, but, as the rate of drug use was several times higher in Harlem than in other boroughs, they could not look away. Dr. Berle wrote, "We soon found out that we could not ignore the drug problem. We were all neighbors. Heroin addicts stole from the clinic as they did from their own families—and if we were truly family physicians, how could we refuse to treat the son of one of our families when he had a boil at the site of an injection made with a dirty needle?"

Then came Marie, offering psychoanalysis and prescribing tranquilizers to help with home detox. Along with a pediatrician, a public health nurse, and a team of social anthropologists, their team performed house calls, bringing evidence-based medicine into communities unfamiliar with such approaches. Before their clinic, parents had no other choice but to carry their sick children through the snow to the nearest hospital. Yet many of Dr. Berle's colleagues thought both she and her novel techniques were crazy. Perhaps it's not surprising that Dr. Berle became a kind of mentor for Marie.[30]

Unfortunately, their results were abysmal. Out of 268 patients who applied to go through a home detox, only 53 actually completed it, and only 10 remained abstinent for at least six months. As Dr. Berle and Marie wrote in their summary paper, "The major difficulties encountered did not lie in the withdrawal procedure but in helping the patient to remain abstinent."[31] And, unfortunately, many of Marie's patients died, young men and women who should have had decades stretching in front of them, talented jazz musicians with brilliant careers yet to be fully realized.

Marie described her resulting sense of despair to Courtwright: "By that time I had exhausted every psychiatric and psychological treatment modality that there was. You name it—hypnosis, group therapy, moving patients around the world, etcetera." Despite her recent breakthroughs in addiction science, and despite the high quality, community-based treatment she was providing, nothing seemed to make a difference. "I was frustrated, very depressed—there was nothing I could do." There had to be a better way.

"Methadone, in a sense, was your salvation," suggested Courtwright. It was 1983, and he and Marie were sitting in her Rockefeller office. Although methadone maintenance had been designed to save those with addiction, it had also saved Marie, just as bupe had saved me.

One afternoon, Marie was venting to a friend of hers who was a medical writer. They were chatting in her living room, which I imagine had tall wooden ceilings and walls lined with bookshelves and modern paintings. Either classical music or jazz was playing, its warm crackles audible on the record player, and they were sitting on a velvet couch, their toes massaged by the luscious rug beneath their feet. As she complained how all her patients inevitably relapsed, he asked her, "Marie, did you ever stop to think what's so wrong about giving the addicts drugs?"[32]

Initially, Marie was so incensed by her friend's suggestion that she almost fainted and kicked him out of her house, although I'm not entirely sure why. Didn't she herself give morphine to her patients at Narco as a Christmas present? In any case, she closed her eyes, took a deep breath, and considered his proposition.

She remembered how Dr. Herbert Berger, one of the other Narcotics Anonymous board members, used to talk about the British approach to heroin addiction. In Britain, addiction was seen as a disease, not a crime, and, thus, its management was left to the medical profession, not law enforcement.[33] Physicians were allowed to treat addiction as they saw fit, even prescribing daily morphine or heroin to those who continued to relapse.

Then there was the book, a weathered copy of the thousand-page tome *The Opium Problem*, that Winick had left on their clinic bookshelf, a book so influential that Anslinger had tried to ban it from public libraries. I could see Marie lifting it, her trim biceps tensing under its hefty weight, and flipping through its fragile, yellowed pages. It was written in 1928 by a husband-and-wife physician team, Charles Terry and Mildred Pellens. In the first chapter, they described the United States' brief experiment with state-sponsored addiction clinics that gave free opioids to users. These clinics were the direct forerunner of today's methadone clinics and, in many ways, even went beyond them, demonstrating that illicit drug traffic decreased when users were allowed to buy their drugs in a safe, regulated environment.[34]

Marie told Courtwright, "You began to get experience when other people more courageous than yourself, and more intelligent, showed you that there were other ways." *The Opium Problem*

helped Marie see America's opioid epidemic as an "an artificial tragedy with real victims" caused by the criminalization of drugs and
addiction.[35] Maybe her friend wasn't so crazy after all.

Beginning to see opioid maintenance as the only path forward,
she told a journalist in 1958, "The proposal to legalize narcotics is
an excellent one. Only when the addict population can come out of
hiding to receive treatment can America hope to come to grips with
this tremendous socio-medical problem."[36] So, by the time she met
Vince in October 1963,[37] she was thoroughly convinced that "the
solution to all the drug problems was to give them more heroin."[38]

CHAPTER 7

Sisyphus

2020

The first time I ordered buprenorphine in the Tucson ED, my Ascom, the bulky portable phone carried by all the nurses and doctors, rang in my pocket. It was the hospital pharmacist. "Are you sure that you meant to order this medication?" he asked.

"Yes," I answered.

"Well, looking at the patient's chart, she doesn't seem to be on this medication."

"That's right. I want to start her on it." I tapped my fingers on my desk, confused by the questioning.

"Ah, I see," he said, his tone revealing his discomfort. "But why are you ordering such a high dose? Eight milligrams seems like a lot. Usually we just do two milligrams at a time for an induction."

I raised my eyebrows—another reminder that I was no longer at Highland, where ordering high doses of bupe had been quick and easy. Later, I would learn that I was even lucky to have bupe in our ED; many hospitals in Southern Arizona, as in much of the country, did not even stock it.

Two hours passed before the medication arrived at the patient's bedside, and the ED resident and nurse were even more flummoxed than the pharmacist. Like me during fellowship, they had never heard of this medication. Leaning against a wall outside the patient's room, I eagerly explained. Now that I had been pulled back into addiction, I couldn't look away, constantly finding more opportunities to make local addiction care better. The passion and purpose I had felt at the startup was back.

A few weeks later, I was standing under the bright lights at the front of a large conference room. "We all know that we are in the middle of an opioid epidemic, so I won't bore you with those statistics," I began, several faces peering down at me from amphitheater seating. I was presenting at the monthly faculty meeting, and I felt a little uncomfortable lecturing to colleagues I didn't yet know. But when I asked our chair if such a talk might be useful for the other attending physicians, he eagerly scheduled the time.

"Instead, I am here to encourage you to begin treatment in the emergency department." I advanced my slide to a table of results. "Typically, we refer patients with chaotic use to outpatient treatment at a methadone clinic. But in 2015, Dr. Gail D'Onofrio's landmark study from Yale showed that doesn't work very well. Thirty days later, only 37 percent of those patients were receiving addiction treatment. In contrast, when the first dose of buprenorphine is given in the emergency department, 78 percent are still enrolled in treatment at thirty days."[1]

Sweat forming on my palms, I paused and looked around the room, wondering what my audience was thinking. Most chewing on sandwiches provided by a local caterer, their expressions gave nothing away.

I launched into buprenorphine's pharmacology. I hoped that if my colleagues realized that buprenorphine was safer than the other opioids we regularly gave, they would feel less skittish about it. I mean, we weren't particularly worried about prescribing full opioids such as Percocet, oxycodone, or Norco. On average, one out of every six patients treated in an emergency department received an opioid prescription.[2] If a patient truly needed an opioid medication for the acute pain of a broken bone or a kidney stone, we would prescribe it.

Yet, in terms of the opioid epidemic, most of us ED docs thought our paltry prescribing absolved us from any blame. Although we wrote a lot of prescriptions for opioids, they were for small quantities, just enough to get someone through a few a days of excruciating pain.[3] We didn't think that fifteen pills here or there were enough to get anyone addicted. But a study by Dr. Jason Hoppe questioned that assumption; of opioid-naive patients who received an opioid prescription from the ED, 12 percent went on to recurrent use.[4]

So, if we were regularly prescribing opioids for pain control, even though they could cause further dependence and addiction, why were we so hesitant to start buprenorphine? Bupe was less likely to lead to respiratory depression and fatal overdose and was increasingly considered the first-line of treatment for opioid addiction, a condition we were partially responsible for creating.[5] If we were part of the problem, shouldn't we also be part of the solution?

In one of my most illustrative slides, a red line representing fatal overdoses plummeted as a green line representing patients on MOUD climbed skyward. When France expanded access almost fivefold to methadone and buprenorphine between 1996 and 2003, deaths dropped by almost the same amount.[6] Same thing in Baltimore.[7]

Patients receiving MOUD were also more likely to remain engaged in addiction treatment. In Sweden, a group of scientists, including Dr. Mary Jeanne Kreek, randomized forty patients with opioid use disorder to either receive daily buprenorphine for twelve months or a tapered six-day regimen of daily buprenorphine followed by a placebo.[8] In addition, volunteers in both arms received cognitive behavioral group therapy and weekly individual counseling, so the psychosocial support they were receiving was a lot more robust than what most people have access to.

In the placebo group, every single patient dropped out of addiction treatment by two months. In contrast, 75 percent of the patients on daily buprenorphine were still in treatment one year later. The behavioral interventions alone were not enough to keep the participants engaged in addiction treatment. Furthermore, 20 percent of the placebo group died within the year, whereas everybody in the buprenorphine group survived. Some research suggests that upward of 90 percent of patients in abstinence-based programs relapse, so the results are not particularly surprising. But they are stark.[9]

Even without counseling or behavioral interventions, MOUD seemed to work well. Although behavioral interventions seemed to enhance outcomes for patients receiving methadone, the evidence was less clear for patients taking buprenorphine. In fact, some studies showed no difference in treatment outcomes.[10] Because of this, the American Academy of Emergency Medicine wrote in their opioid use disorder white paper, "providers should not link the initiation of [MOUD] to the immediate availability of or patient willingness to participate in counseling."[11] Yet many did, which meant they were extremely unlikely to start MOUD treatment for any patient in the ED.

My slideshow ended. "Any questions?" I asked.

The room was silent. Perhaps that meant that the evidence was so convincing that there was nothing left to say? The chair of our department thanked me, and I hurried back to my seat.

A few days later, I got my first clue that I was a little off base. I was scrolling through the patient track board in the ED when my colleague arrived for his shift. As nobody wanted to get sick during flu season, he had donned purple gloves and was starting to decon his computer and keyboard with a sanitizing wipe when he turned to ask me, "Are some people on Suboxone forever?"

"Well, ideally people will taper off over a few years, but, yes, some people may be on it forever."

"I guess I just don't see the point of that," he said, his gaze returning to his sanitation procedure. I was too shocked to know what to say. We gave all kinds of medications to people with the expectation that they would likely need them forever, such as those for diabetes, hypertension, or hypothyroidism. How was this any different?

On a different evening, I slid open the glass doors of a patient's room for an evaluation. He was lying in bed, eyes shut, as two nurses leaned over his arms looking for veins. His lower leg was beefy red and hot to the touch, signs consistent with the resident's diagnosis of a cellulitis caused by reusing syringes. But when I asked the resident if the patient was experiencing withdrawal, she didn't know. She hadn't asked about that.

I thought this was a serious omission. According to his medical record, he was last admitted several months ago for a similar condition, but he left after only twenty-four hours, just around the time when the pains of withdrawal became too much to bear. Because he was not offered treatment, he left the hospital to use before he could receive the antibiotics that he needed to heal. Unfortunately, he was not unique. Patients with a substance use disorder are three times more likely to leave the hospital against medical advice (AMA) than others.[12] This number is even higher for patients who inject drugs; in one study, 25 percent left AMA.[13]

Yet, just as I had not initially regretted how I treated my "drug-seeking" patient during residency, this young man's doctors probably did not feel any personal responsibility for his AMA discharge. Instead of seeing his early departure as a consequence of their inadequate medical treatment, they likely believed he just wasn't as serious about his health as they were. Even the term "against medical advice" made it sound like the patient's fault.

After I introduced myself, I asked him, "Do you feel like you're experiencing any withdrawal? I just ask because I want to let you know that we have medications that can help you."

He turned his brown eyes away from the nurse at his forearm to meet my gaze. "No, but, what do you have?"

"Methadone and Suboxone. Have you tried either?"

He nodded. "Yeah, Suboxone."

"Did it work well for you?"

"Yeah. I'd like that again," he answered.

"Did you get it from a clinic or the streets?"

"The street." If we weren't going to help him, he would find people who would. A study out of North Carolina showed that so-called "diverted" buprenorphine was used correctly most of the time, with people using it when experiencing withdrawal. It also showed that the biggest cause of diverted buprenorphine was substantial barriers to legal access. Because it didn't offer a high, and because the euphoric fentanyl was so widely available, it was unlikely to be abused by opioid-naive people. In fact, I had never heard of that happening.

I continued: "Okay, well, just let us know when you start to feel sick. Unlike methadone, you have to already be sick before you can start Suboxone, otherwise it will make you feel worse. But we have it in the hospital and can start it when you're ready." He nodded silently.[14]

Back in the doc box, hip-hop playing over the speakers, I found the resident sitting at a row of computers on the back wall of the square-shaped room. I told her about the conversation I had with the patient, and she agreed to tell the admitting hospitalist team about our plan.

I cautioned, "They probably aren't familiar with how to start Suboxone, so you should probably spell it out for them."

I gave her instructions, just in case she wasn't familiar with the procedure, either. I wanted to make it easy for them. The resident nodded and returned to work.

Thinking everything was taken care of, I moved on to think about the plans for my other patients: a man whose dental infection had spread to his chest wall, a woman who was bleeding out of a wound in her abdomen, a man with what the lay press called "flesh-eating bacteria." I was also stuffing a spring roll into my mouth, as there were no "dinner breaks" in the ED. But when I overheard the resident having a stilted conversation over the phone, I paused my chewing to listen more carefully.

She was clutching the gray plastic phone to her ear, presumably talking to the hospitalist who would soon be caring for our man with the cellulitis. She said, "Umm, well, that's the advice my attending gave me."

I had heard this before; it meant she was getting some pushback that she didn't know how to respond to.

After a pause to listen to the hospitalist, she continued, "She said that we do have buprenorphine in the hospital."

I walked over to her swivel chair, extending my palm. "Can I talk to the doc?" I asked.

"Here, my attending wants to talk to you." She raised her eyebrows and handed over the phone.

"Hi, this is Dr. Glenn. I heard you had a question about starting buprenorphine?" I tried to sound friendly and nonthreatening, to prevent my voice from betraying the frustration I felt.

"Oh, hi, yes, I mean, I don't want to argue or anything," the hospitalist started. "And I'm not the doctor who will ultimately be taking care of him. I'm just getting the report and then assigning him to another hospitalist."

"That's okay!" I responded. "I'm still happy to answer any questions about buprenorphine, since this will probably come up again." I took a sip of water.

"Our division chief has said that we can't start buprenorphine without a waiver," she said. At the time, a special x-waiver from the DEA was needed to prescribe buprenorphine, but not to start it in the hospital.

"Luckily, that's not true!" I gesticulated with my free hand, even though the doc on the other end couldn't see. "I can send you the code of federal regulations document that explains how inpatient teams, as long as they are admitting a patient for something other than addiction—in this case, a soft tissue infection—can start MOUD, even without a waiver."

She said, "Like I said, I'm not the doc taking care of him, and I've heard from our chief that you can't."

I sighed. Nothing I said would convince her otherwise. Although she could not tell me what specific regulation prohibited buprenorphine, she still clung to this anecdotal tidbit she had heard at some point. This was exactly the intended effect of confusing regulation: make it so the doctors didn't want to get involved. Make avoidance so much easier.

Twenty minutes later, I had a similar conversation with the hospitalist who would ultimately be responsible for this man's care. He was more blunt: "Look, a Sunday night is not the time for education."

My mouth opened into a little "o."

He continued: "I'm behind in all the work that I have to get done in time for tomorrow—clearance for cardiac caths and procedures, not to mention my admissions."

Hearing the harried tone in his voice, I began to feel a little more sympathetic.

"Can you get an addiction medicine consult?" he asked.

"Sure," I answered.

After the call ended, I typed up the instructions in a carefully detailed note. Dr. Elissa Gumm had recently started an addiction medicine consult service at our hospital, and, although it wasn't available on Sunday nights, I was one of the docs allowed to write notes for them. I did not really have time to do it, as I was supervising several residents caring for about twenty patients, some of them critically ill, but if this is what it took for my patient to get his medication, I was going to do it. I had just read a study authored by a colleague of mine in San Francisco, Dr. Hannah Snyder, showing that inpatients started on MOUD were more than three times as likely to continue treatment after discharge. This was our opportunity.

However, the next day at work, when I logged into this patient's chart to follow his progress, I saw a note from the hospitalist in which he had written, "As I do not have an x-waiver, I cannot start buprenorphine."

Why had I bothered to write the consult note if he was unwilling to listen? Anger pulsed through my fingertips and up to my face. Once again, I was coming up against these erroneous beliefs. Of course, it wasn't the ignorance and misinformation that bothered me, as I knew firsthand how little this material was covered during our medical training. It was the lack of the willingness to learn.

Even when I tried to make it easy, explaining the regulations word for word, it seemed like doctors rarely believed me.[15] Was it because I was young? A woman? Or just because something about treating addiction felt untoward, suspicious? Vestiges of a century of criminalization? Stigma? Of course, it didn't help that the regulations were so confusing, that the permission to give MOUD was buried deep in the Federal Register.

Initially, I just tried harder to educate the nonbelievers. I sent scientific papers. I sent position statements from various professional organizations. I sent documents that explained the tangled laws around MOUD. I offered to speak at their faculty meetings. I connected them to other addiction specialists, hoping that maybe they would believe someone else. But for the people who were staunchly anti-MOUD, none of this seemed to work. The resistance was not lodged in their brains, but in their hearts.

I felt like a young Marie, fighting the whole system by myself. Of course, my frustration was nothing like that felt daily by people who used, marginalized every step of the way. But, still, I was exhausted. I knew that changing culture and practice took time, but it was time we didn't have. Every day, we lost more people to senseless overdoses. I remembered the haggard tone of Christopher's voice during his naloxone training, the one that I initially found off-putting. Now I understood.

Unfortunately, it wasn't just my colleagues who saw MOUD through a lens of stigma; it was also my patients and their families. One of my patients at the methadone clinic was a young man with a lot of ambition and drive. Our appointments were late in the afternoon so as not to interfere with his job in construction, and his clothes were always a little dusty when he arrived; he had no time to shower between work and clinic close.

The week after he started bupe, he told me he felt great. Even though he was only taking a low dose, he didn't have any cravings, and he hadn't used. For the first time in years, he felt normal. Over the weekend, he and his wife took the kids horseback riding. This was exactly how buprenorphine was supposed to work. But then he asked something that worried me: "Can you tell me how to taper off this stuff?"

I paused, turning away from my keyboard to face him, hands clasped in my lap. "Well, we usually recommend that patients stay on MOUD for at least two years before stopping. It takes time to get your life stable again, to allow the neuroplasticity of your brain to reroute your neuropathways around pain and reward."

He was sitting on the vinyl couch against the window, shades drawn. He looked straight at me. "I can't wait that long. If my wife knows I'm on this, she is going to leave me. She is going to take the kids and leave."

"But why?" I asked. "Buprenorphine is treatment."

"Yeah, well," he waved his hand in the air. "She doesn't think that way."

"Would it help if I called her?" I asked, a hopeful tone creeping into my voice.

He leaned forward, eyes opening wide. "No, no, please don't do that. In fact, are there any settings you can note in my chart about this? I don't want any calls from this number, or anything mailed to my home address. She can't know."

I turned to my computer, and, sure enough, there was such a setting for me to click. I just hoped it wasn't too late. Facing him again, I continued, "I have seen too many people relapse when they quit their medications before two years. Just as we do with any other chronic condition, we don't rush to discontinue treatments if they are working. For example, we don't ask diabetics to quit taking their insulin. Instead, we are happy that we found a dose that finally worked."

Then I repeated a line that I had heard from one of Courtwright's interviews: "If a man had a below-the-knee amputation, and you gave him a prosthetic leg, would you encourage him to stop using it as soon as possible, referring to it as a crutch? Of course not. Most Americans have some chronic condition for which they take medication. Addiction is no different."[16]

He was unwavering. "I will be different. I won't relapse. You'll see."

My heart sank. I hoped he was right, but I had seen too many people say the same thing and fail. Additionally, the data supported my concern. The next week, he didn't come to our scheduled appointment. Nor the week after that. I hoped it was because he was doing well, not because he was dead. I'll never know.

CHAPTER 8

The Cure

1965

The year was 1965. I imagine Marie sitting next to Vincent at the kitchen table, drinking her morning coffee and smoking a cigarette, when this month's issue of *JAMA*, one of the most prestigious medical journals in the world, landed on their doorstep. Marie and Vince exchanged a grin and flipped immediately to their groundbreaking article, "A Medical Treatment for Diacetylmorphine (Heroin) Addiction." Marie gave a small leap. "Look, Vince, we did it!" Laughter bubbled from her throat. "The Bureau of Narcotics tried to shut us down, but we showed them."

This publication was the fruit of over two years of labor, one that they believed would change the future of heroin addiction forever. They had found a treatment that worked: methadone. Although methadone itself was nothing new, their concept was. Instead of using methadone as a treatment for acute pain, or as a temporary medication to help someone detox off opioids, they were giving high doses every day, indefinitely, in the form of maintenance treatment. For the first time, they were suggesting that an opioid-free existence did not need to be the goal of addiction treatment. To many, this was heretical. Also illegal. Ever since the 1919 Supreme Court case *Webb v. United States*, using opioids in the form of maintenance treatment for addiction had been prohibited.

Although Marie had been working in addiction for almost twenty years when she joined Vince's lab in 1962, Vince was an accidental newcomer to the field. Prior to the 1960s, he was a metabolic disease researcher studying hypertension and obesity. But he wasn't just anybody. As Marie put it, he was respected by the people whose opinion mattered, by the people in the "top echelons of medicine" in a way that she was not: leaders at the National Institutes of Health, deans of prestigious medical schools, and established researchers. One of their colleagues claimed he was on track to win a Nobel Prize for his metabolic research.[1]

During Vince's daily commute from Rye to Manhattan, he passed through Harlem, a community then facing high rates of crime and heroin addiction. He described it as "moving between two highly privileged oases through a truly epidemic sea of misery." He told Courtwright: "I began to realize that nobody in my community of scientists or people in Rye had any concept of that world. We were essentially living in the midst of an epidemic and ignoring it."[2] One of Vince's colleagues happened to be the chair of the city's Health Research Council Committee on Narcotics and was looking to pass the role onto someone else. When Vince lamented to him about the dearth of medical and pharmaceutical research in addiction, he knew he had found his replacement.

As the new chair, Vincent figured he should learn something about addiction, so he read all the literature, consulted all the leading experts, and even visited Narco. But Marie's approach was the only one that made any sense to him. Vince devoured her 1956 book, *The Drug Addict as a Patient*, in which she posited that addiction was a medical disease, not a crime in need of incarceration, and made the radical claims that patients should enter treatment of their own accord instead of being forced by the carceral system, doctors should not abandon their patients who wished to only cut down on their use instead of quitting, and maintenance treatment with morphine and heroin should be considered a viable option for some users.[3]

When Vince called Marie for advice, she demurred that she wasn't the one he needed to talk to; these were questions he should be asking the patients themselves. When he agreed to meet her at the city's only detox and rehabilitation units, I imagine Marie leading the way as they ascended Metropolitan Hospital's elevator to the fifteenth floor, the skirt of her A-line dress swinging as they walked.[4] When residents and patients saw Marie, their faces brightened. "Hi Doc!" a young man exclaimed. "I was listening to Charlie Parker yesterday and it made me think of you. Have you been out to any good shows?"

Marie's warm laugh echoed in the cavernous hallway of the Art Deco building. "Oh, I wish, but I've been spending all my time here with you! Should we play a little duet later?"

Marie's gusto and easy rapport with patients and staff captivated Vince. He told Courtwright, "She impressed me as a very intense and intelligent person who was working under absolutely hopeless disadvantages administratively. She was all alone, with a good heart and a lot of spirit, trying to fight the establishment up and down the line."[5]

Their conversation continued over several more lunches and meetings, and pretty soon he asked if she would work with him. He wanted to better understand what users actually looked like on drugs, as he did not believe it had ever been appropriately studied. Although the pharmacology of various opioids had been studied at the Narco Farm in Lexington, he envisioned something more applicable to real life. I imagine that Marie met this proposal with shock—how would he do such a thing?—and a little rebellious excitement. As the bureau didn't even like the fact that she was providing outpatient talk therapy to addicts, how would they respond to the even more radical act of administering narcotics?

Perhaps he then leaned in over their lunch table at a New York deli, cocking one eyebrow higher than the other, pulling his thick lips to the side in a way that showed the dimple in his cheek, and said, "I'm not going to ask for permission."

Dr. Robert Newman, a physician who followed Marie and Vincent's lead to create the world's largest methadone maintenance program in 1970 New York, explained to Courtwright how important this approach was for the future of methadone maintenance, how it allowed Marie and Vincent to "unequivocally win the battle" for methadone against the Bureau of Narcotics: "I think if they had simply submitted a written request to the bureaucracy and made all kinds of appeals to get permission to do what they intended to do, I don't think today we'd have any methadone programs. I think they just made the decision that they were going to go ahead and do it. And they were subjected to tremendous harassment and threats as a result of this, but had they waited, in other words, if the federal bureaucracy had been able to decide in a vacuum whether or not to permit this kind of treatment, it would have been very easy for the government to maintain the status quo and simply say *no, this is not acceptable.* . . . So you know, I think they [won the battle] through sheer courage in terms of doing what they thought was right."[6]

But Vincent was not stupid. Although he had not asked the Bureau of Narcotics for permission, he did ask the Rockefeller Institute. If they endorsed his controversial research, it would be the institute who was giving drugs to addicts, not just "two kooky doctors."[7] He also won approval from leading medical organizations, providing a much broader base of support. As Vince was friends with many of the physicians who held distinguished positions in America's house of medicine, he was easily able to convince them of the scientific merit of and need for such investigation. In addition, Vincent persuaded the City of New York's Health Research Council to fund them, adding even more legitimacy.

Marie was impressed by his connections and political savvy, and, of course, by the idea itself. Vincent found her at just the right time, when her frustration had reached a feverish peak. In her mind, there was only one thing left to try—and now, in the name of science, she would finally be able to do it.

Initially, Marie and Vincent started with just two patients: two men who were addicted to heroin. For the duration of the study, they lived in a dedicated ward at the Rockefeller Institute and were cared for by a cadre of nurses and staff trained by Marie. Initially, the goal was just to keep the men comfortable, so they were given various narcotics. But Marie quickly realized it "was an impossible task." As I listened to her describe the scenario to David Courtwright, the scene started to unroll in my mind.

The historic ward felt spacious, with tall vaulted ceilings and tiled floors, and, instead of individual rooms, patient beds were separated by beige curtains. In the center, a waist-high counter in the shape of a square demarcated the central nursing station. Leaning against it, Marie scribbled an order in one of the patient's charts for morphine. The patient's nurse drew up the clear liquid into a glass syringe and went to find the young man, who, at this point, had the sweaty forehead, dilated pupils, and goosebumps typical of withdrawal. She squeezed his deltoid between the fingers of her left hand and plunged the needle into his muscle.

Although relief passed over his face, it did not last long. One hour later and he was already begging the nurse for more. The two men never got comfortable and always seemed to be watching the clock, aware of the exact time they could ask for their next dose. After a while, they stopped getting dressed. Not only that, but the amount of morphine they needed to feel somewhat normal continued to escalate. First it was just four milligrams, then six, then eight. Where would it stop? Watching them, Marie sighed as her frustration returned. They didn't seem to have "any goals other than waiting for the next shot." She tried various drugs: heroin, morphine, Dilaudid, cough medicine, everything she'd ever heard of, but none of it worked. Perhaps agonist treatment with opioids wasn't the answer, either.

Before giving up, they decided to try one last thing: methadone. At this point, the men were on high doses of opioids, so they had to use equivalently high doses of methadone: eighty, ninety, one hundred milligrams. Marie was scared to give such an amount, as it was unprecedented; she had never heard of anyone giving a dose higher than forty milligrams, and that was just for the temporary management of getting someone through the agony of withdrawals. But higher doses seemed necessary to overcome their cravings and physiologic dependence, so that was what they did.

And then something remarkable happened. When she returned to the hospital ward the next day, the two patients were "unlike anything that we had previously seen; their color was good, they weren't thinking of drugs, they wanted to go to school—it was clear they were ready for rehabilitation." At first, she thought it was all an illusion, a false hope. As she told Courtwright, "I had been around too long and seen too many miracles which turned out not to work." But a young intern that they had recently hired to help with data collection, Dr. Mary Jean Kreek, convinced her it was real. In her documentation, Kreek wrote how the men were requesting to go to school and wanted to find jobs. Seeing the staggering results written there, on paper, Marie almost collapsed.

Marie kept them on their daily methadone, and, unlike with the other opioids, their doses did not escalate. Although she and Vincent looked for evidence of adverse side effects, they found none. They even brought in psychologists to measure if the men's response times were delayed, but they were not. For the first time in years, the men felt *normal*.

Still, when the men started to leave the ward at night to attend night school, Marie worried. Although she knew that methadone worked just fine within the locked confines of a hospital, what about on the streets? What about when they passed friends who were using? What then? She stopped going home, instead waiting "in total terror" until they returned.

One night, Marie was nearly asleep in a corner chair when the men swung open the ward's heavy door. They waved their hellos and came closer, each innocently licking an ice cream cone. On their walk home from class, they had run into some guys shooting heroin, but, instead of feeling tempted, they stopped and bought some ice cream. They laughed at this surprising scenario, nobody happier than they. Marie smiled so wide her cheeks hurt.

As Marie and Vincent added more patients to their study, it wasn't long before the Bureau of Narcotics got wind of what they were up to. An agent stormed over to the Rockefeller Institute, banging on the ward's locked doors and demanding to be let inside. He looked official enough, wearing a trench coat like you might see in any detective series on TV, and so the nurse let him in. He then marched right into Vincent's office, slammed his hands down on the desk Vincent was working on, leaned his face closer, and shouted, "You're breaking the law!"[8]

Vincent calmly put down his pen and stood up, his tall, wide frame now almost towering. Slowly, weighing every word, he replied, "Well, I've been looking into that, and, as far as I understand it, I'm not."

Not used to such defiance, the agent's eyes opened wide. "You are!" His voice started to become shrill. "If you don't stop, we'll put you out of business."

Vincent was undeterred. "Maybe that's the proper thing to do. The thing you ought to do, given the way you understand it, is to sue me." In preparation for such a confrontation, Vincent had already gone to Rockefeller's attorneys, who had drawn up an exhaustive legal brief that basically concluded that, despite the bureau's assertions, there actually existed no substantive law prohibiting the research that Marie and Vincent were planning. The Harrison Act stated that physicians were allowed to administer opioids "in the course of medical practice," and if they were giving maintenance opioids in the course of state-sponsored research, shouldn't that be considered legitimate medical practice?

The agent's face dropped in shock, and, without further discussion, he turned to leave. But this would not be the last that Marie and Vincent saw of the Bureau of Narcotics. Vince explained, "They assigned agents to monitor everything that we did, and to come with various threats to us, saying that we were not doing things that were bona fide and we better watch out." But once the bureau realized that outright attacks wouldn't scare Vince and Marie, they changed their methods.

Vince told Courtwright, "They infiltrated clinics and stole records in order to get what they considered inside information, and they leaked out or encouraged various kinds of attacks on us, and floated various rumors that had to do with our activities that weren't true and did what they could to discredit us with legislators and various other bodies to try to encourage them to set up prohibiting legislation, and they even were very active with the National Research Council, trying to get that prestigious body to condemn our work, so they shifted their tactic from outright attack to attempts to discredit us. Really quite remarkably."

In the end, this is how the bureau would win, through public fear-mongering and the promulgation of legal barriers, how methadone would never be given a chance to be successful. With less than 2 percent of American physicians offering MOUD, perhaps it is no surprise that we are living in the midst of our country's worst opioid epidemic yet. Every day, over one hundred Americans die of an opioid overdose, far more than the number dying from car accidents or guns. Opioid overdose is now the seventh most frequent cause of death.[9] Despite the increasingly common rhetoric heard these days about how addiction is now seen as a disease, by and large our country and its physicians still are not treating it as such.

But, of course, Marie and Vincent couldn't know all that. They only saw the transformative potential of methadone maintenance, and once they had results from twenty-two subjects, they decided it was time to collate their results and share them with the world. The longer they waited to share this treatment, the more people would die. I imagine it was around this time that Vincent realized that he would never be returning to his metabolic research, and that Marie and Vincent started to fall in love, even though they were both already married. The passion for their work blurred into a passion for each other, and late nights at the hospital turned into an affair. The year 1965 wasn't just when their study was published in *JAMA*; it was also the year that Marie and Vincent divorced their spouses and married each other.

CHAPTER 9

Hope

2021

"Our naloxone program is finally here!" I shouted over the din of the ED dox box chatter. The residents and attendings swiveled in their chairs to see. I set the clear plastic container in the middle of the counter, opened the latch, and pulled out a pink and white cardboard box of naloxone as I instructed, "Give one to anyone who might be at risk of an opioid overdose! Anyone and everyone. We have plenty more where this came from."

After over a year of stagnation, our distribution program had finally been approved. Just as Marie and Vince had learned, barriers often seemed to appear when it came to helping people who used drugs. But, instead of letting them stop you, the trick was to go around them, and now I was on a first-name basis with leadership at the Arizona State Board of Pharmacy and the Arizona Department of Health Services. Furthermore, the Department of Health hoped I could help expand this program across the state.

"While you're here," one of the residents asked, "can I ask you a buprenorphine question?"

I grinned and pulled up a chair. "Of course!"

A small circle of residents scooted closer to listen, and the attending proudly told me that he just applied for his DEA-x to prescribe buprenorphine. Lately, more of my colleagues had been interested in starting MOUD, and it was not uncommon for them to call me with clinical questions. Whereas I normally dreaded work calls during the weekends and evenings, I happily answered when it was about MOUD.

Lately, I was even starting to recommend that my colleagues start methadone instead of buprenorphine, going against the bupísta dogma I had embraced at Highland. After working several months at the methadone clinic, I now agreed with Dr. Oñate that methadone really was the better option for some. Many of my patients enjoyed coming to the clinic every day, the routine and accountability supporting their recovery. Some liked methadone because it worked better to control their cravings, and others preferred it because it was easier to still get high on the weekends. What business of mine was it if my patients still wanted to use? Wasn't my primary goal to support any positive change? As such, I would use that opportunity to advise them how to reduce their risk of overdose, but I wouldn't scold them or cut off their access to methadone. Like many harm reductionists, I was coming to see methadone as a version of safer supply.

Then Chris Edwards, our ED pharmacist, walked into the doc box. His blue eyes sparkled through his glasses. "Are we going to start bupe on someone?" he asked, rubbing his palms together. "Maybe the patient who got Narcan in the field?" Thanks to him, bupe had been stocked in the ED Pyxis machines, meaning it could be given within minutes instead of the hours it used to take to come from the hospital pharmacy. He had also trained a cadre of pharmacy students and residents on addiction treatment. Lately, I no longer felt quite so alone.

Yet, no matter how much we supported our individual patients, larger forces threatened to undo all our efforts: stigmatizing hospital policies that led to harassment, pharmacies refusing to fill prescriptions, insurance companies requiring prior authorizations for life-saving medications as a cost-containment strategy, or laws prohibiting harm reduction. If we truly wanted to help the most vulnerable, we couldn't just stay at the bedside—we would have to change the system itself.

"Also," he added, "our pharmacy resident is interested in doing research related to opioids. Maybe we can work together?"

I beamed with excitement and rubbed my belly, now about five months pregnant with my second daughter. Although I had worried that I had lost my chance to innovate when I left the startup, academics was providing another path, one that felt even more genuine. Soon, one of our research studies would even be published in a national medical journal. I felt like I was following in Marie's footsteps.

In the spring of 2021, the psychiatry chair suggested that we prepare a press release about the addiction services our hospital now offered. When I saw all our accomplishments written down on paper, hopeful pride bubbled in my chest. Little by little, we were making a difference, yet we still had so far to go. Perhaps the press could provide the additional momentum we needed to get there. If patients started to show up in our ED asking for MOUD, newspaper in hand, my skeptical colleagues would have a harder time sweeping addiction under the rug. It would legitimize my claim that addiction treatment was a standard part of emergency medicine.

Additionally, it would help users navigate the confusing treatment landscape. Few local EDs or hospitals gave out naloxone or started MOUD, so it was important to let people know that we did. Some hospitals didn't even offer methadone to admitted patients who had been stable on methadone for years, forcing patients to check out AMA if they wanted their medication. A statement also felt like an opportunity for atonement; in the past, we degraded people who used drugs and sent them away empty-handed. Now we would treat them with humanity and offer real treatments. At least many of us would.

For weeks, we drafted and revised various iterations of our statement. We received approval from the chairs and directors of various departments. Finally, once it was ready, we sent it to the hospital CEOs for one last stamp of approval. I thought we'd be in the press within one to two days. And, although it was no *New York Times*, the site of many of Marie's features, I felt like she would be proud.

CHAPTER 10

Zenith

1960s–1970s

It was around 1963 or 1964, right after Vince and Marie realized that methadone was the future. In my mind, Vince was wearing a dark suit and had a portfolio of documents tucked under his arm as he walked up the concrete steps and passed under the intricate metalwork that highlighted the front doors of the NYC Department of Health. He had an appointment with Dr. Ray Trussell, the commissioner who oversaw all the city's public hospitals. When he opened the door to his office, Dr. Trussell was behind a stack of papers toppling over his walnut desk. His dark hair was cut short, except for the top, which was starting to bald along the edges, and his chin had the slightest dimple. "Come in," he said, his voice softer than Vince had imagined.

"How can I help you today?" Dr. Trussell asked.

Vince was prepared to start from the beginning, to explain why the hospital commissioner should even care about addiction when he had a thousand other diseases clamoring for his attention, but Dr. Trussell already knew. A few years prior, he had asked administrators to dedicate twenty-five of the system's twenty-one thousand beds for pregnant women with addiction. They refused—they didn't want those kinds of patients.[1]

Vince moved on to their trial. "All six patients participating in our methadone program stayed off heroin and returned to work and school." He opened a manila folder and passed some figures and tables over to Dr. Trussell before explaining their clinical protocols.

Dr. Trussell squinted to confirm the numbers. Although it was a small study, a 100 percent success rate was unheard of in addiction medicine, or, for that matter, for any chronic disease.

Vince continued: "Obviously, six patients is not a big enough sample size to really prove anything. We need to enroll more patients. Unfortunately, Rockefeller doesn't have any more beds. I'm wondering if the city could spare six more." Vince leaned in over folded palms.

Dr. Trussell rested the pad of his finger against his round nose, thinking through how he could make this work in the face of such opposition. Finally, he spoke. "Okay. Let's have you speak to the board at Beth Israel."[2]

They said yes.

After those patients showed equally positive results, it was now Dr. Trussell asking the favor. "Vince," he said, his voice crackling over the phone, "we need to get this treatment out there. But to really do that, we need to expand even more. We need to go big."

Although he knew it would be challenging, Vince understood this was the only way forward. To garner support, Trussell invited the mayor, police commissioners, and journalists to see Marie and Vince's operation. Because none of the visitors could distinguish between who was a patient and who was an employee, these site visits were particularly effective in building public support for methadone, much more so than abstract statistics. Almost overnight, the whole thing took off. Trussell asked the mayor's office for $1 million and got it. Then the health department and Beth Israel chipped in. In the summer of 1965,[3] NYC's mayor stood in front of a crowd to announce the methadone demonstration project that Vince would lead at Beth Israel Medical Center and expand to several other municipal hospitals.[4] But it still wasn't enough to meet the city's demand, and their waitlist grew longer and longer.

To unequivocally prove methadone's value, Dr. Trussell formed an evaluation committee led by one of his epidemiology students, Dr. Frances Rowe Gearing. To ensure that their results were legitimate and free of bias, he included members whose beliefs spanned a wide range. If he could get some of methadone's fiercest critics to admit that it worked, perhaps he could win over the city's loudest critics. And loud they were. Even the director of the city's own Addiction Services Agency was staunchly opposed to methadone.[5] At the time, the abstinence-based therapeutic communities were methadone's main competitor, a movement most notoriously represented by a California organization that would later be denounced as a cult: Synanon. Much like today's Narcotics Anonymous, therapeutic communities preached that methadone was just a Band-Aid.[6] As the wife of Synanon's East Coast director told a *New York Times* journalist, "Methadone is just substituting one drug for another, and I think that's criminal. Drug addicts can be cured without taking any drugs. The proof is here in Synanon."[7]

Initially, Trussell's evaluation committee faced resistance from Marie and her right-hand woman, Dr. Joyce Lowinson. Joyce was a slim, petite woman with a wide smile who had worked under Marie as a psychiatry resident. During Joyce's senior year, Marie asked her to join their Rockefeller lab. Over the years that followed, Joyce would direct the new unit at Beth Israel, open more clinics, and become the founding director of Einstein's Division of Substance Abuse. Like Marie, Joyce had never envisioned a career in addiction, instead planning to become a psychiatry professor. But something about Marie changed her mind.

Her voice quavering in the way typical of a woman in her nineties, Joyce told me, "I wasn't the first to fall in love with her upon her first meeting. She was a very warm, funny, and bright woman. It was instantaneous." I could relate. Before long, Joyce was one of Marie's closest friends. When Marie divorced Leonard and moved out of their apartment, it was Joyce and Marie's mom who cleaned out her things. When Marie married Vince, Joyce was her bridesmaid.

When Dr. Frances Gearing showed up in the hospital to collect data on the female patients receiving methadone, Joyce and Marie met her at the door. "They were very reluctant to let us get any information about the women," Dr. Gearing said, her voice deepened by decades of smoking.[8] When she asked Joyce and Marie where the patients' records were located, they shrugged their shoulders. Did she leave that day in a huff, frustrated by the obstacles they were putting in her path?

Dr. Gearing would later learn that they hid the records on "little pieces of paper in their pocketbooks," as they did not trust her with their patients' secrets. Many had been prostitutes, a few were lesbians, and they didn't want that information to get to the press. Of course, that wasn't what Dr. Gearing was interested in. "That was probably one of the worst roadblocks we had . . . by virtue of two very strong women. . . . As it turned out, they became two of my greatest supporters later on, but at the beginning, they were rough. . . . It was a rough fight."[9]

Dr. Gearing added, "Now remember, they were harassed from all sides on the fact that they were giving this horrible thing": methadone. And when Marie and Vince began to study female patients, the FDA was "on their backs all the time." Women were seen by the public as vulnerable and precious, worthy of paternalistic protection. For this reason, drug trials often excluded women back then, just as they exclude pregnant and breastfeeding women today. Yet, as we all know, these "precious" women still get sick and take medications, just without the benefit of knowing whether they are safe or not. And, of course, women also become addicted to heroin.

In 1967, Dr. Gearing's committee shared their evaluation with the city, and, the next day, *The New York Times* ran the story. Out of the 383 patients studied, 78 percent were able to hold jobs, go to school, or do both with the help of methadone maintenance. Dr. Gearing said of her evaluation, "Everybody wanted it to come out to be no good. . . . They wanted a report saying this was just another one of those pies in the sky. . . . I can tell you the first three reports I brought out, nobody believed 'em except those who wanted to," a deep laugh crept into her voice, "who already believed! There was a point in that whole thing where I was sure I was beating my head against a stone wall."[10]

That was exactly how I felt when trying to convince many of my colleagues to use methadone and buprenorphine. Although

I was presenting to physicians who should be swayed by robust studies and data, the research never seemed to change their minds. I kept collecting more papers, showing them more citations, but it didn't make a bit of difference. I wondered if a story would make the difference in a way that numbers could not, as it could appeal to something more emotional. The French Marxist philosopher Louis Althusser suggested that texts are one of the primary ways in which people shape their identities.[11] When a text hails us, we turn around as when we hear a familiar voice in the street. There is a sense of recognition, of being seen. After all, it was a story at a book club that hailed me. Could a story about methadone and Marie do the same for others?

In a 1983 interview, Dr. Gearing said that this project was "probably the biggest challenge I ever had in my life, and I enjoyed rising to the bit because I had firm confidence in the fact that I knew what I was talking about, and this makes it very comfortable." She laughed. "Sometimes, you get involved in controversy and you're not quite sure if you are right or not, but in this situation, I knew I was right, and I felt great confidence. At times I enjoyed the controversy. It got a little exhausting at times," her words again broken by a chuckle, "I used to get a little bit tired." I knew what she meant.

In 1968, Dr. Gearing's results were published in *JAMA*, marking a milestone for methadone's credibility.[12] It didn't come a moment too soon. Crime, drugs, racial tension, hippies, and Vietnam had all coalesced into an electric sense of crisis that hung over New York City and the country at large. Heroin use was increasing, with an estimated one hundred thousand addicts in the city.[13] Hippies were smoking marijuana and burning draft cards. Black nationalists were marching and demanding faster change. The summer of 1967 even received a special name, "The Long, Hot Summer of 1967," because so many race riots erupted across the United States. White America felt like the country was falling apart, and Mayor Lindsay faced intense pressure to do something.[14] Further raising the stakes was the fact that Mayor Lindsay planned to run for president against Richard Nixon, a Republican who portrayed himself as the candidate who would bring stability to a tumultuous time.

What we needed, Nixon argued, was more police. Instead of condemning a criminal for breaking the law, the Democrats criticized society, and their leniency allowed crime to flourish. Nixon ran his campaign on "law and order," which he hoped would also appeal to the South. Until the 1960s, the South had traditionally voted for Democratic candidates. Although Nixon could not directly appeal to Southern voters on issues of white supremacy, he could do so indirectly through the coded, anti-Black rhetoric of support for "states' rights" and "law and order."[15] In more modern terms, he promised to make America great again. In 1968, Nixon won the election, his "Southern strategy" paying off.

Yet, politically, Nixon could not just arrest his way out of addiction, as the face of addiction was changing from Black men in Harlem to white suburbanites, innocent teenagers, and soldiers returning from Vietnam.[16] When up to 20 percent of servicemen in Vietnam suffered from addiction, heroin changed from a problem isolated to "those people" to one that the country cared about fighting.[17] Suddenly, incarceration-as-treatment seemed less popular when it applied to white middle-class kids and veterans.

In the fall of 1970, Mayor Lindsay again stood at city hall, this time announcing the doubling of the city's methadone project.[18] Within a few months, twenty new centers would open across the city, making theirs the largest methadone maintenance program in the world. He had officially chosen methadone over abstinence—a huge boon for addiction treatment. Soon, Nixon would arrive at the same decision. Although Lindsay was a Democrat and Nixon was a Republican, they could agree on one thing: methadone.

At the time, Washington, DC, was known as the crime capital of the nation, and local leaders demanded that Nixon make good on his promises. Could methadone be a cheap solution? Although abstinence-based therapeutic communities might have been more politically favorable, none of them could provide any data about recidivism. They had refused to let Dr. Gearing, or anybody else, study them.[19] In contrast, methadone docs had pages of statistics about recidivism, employment, substance use, and crime that they shared with White House staffers.[20]

In 1968, *JAMA* published a study by Marie and Vince claiming that methadone reduced crime: "The number of criminal addicts who have been rehabilitated with methadone treatment is large enough to empty a moderate sized jail, and there are at least 1,000 more addicts waiting for treatment."[21] Although a more progressive article might suggest that the decriminalization—or better yet, the legalization—of drugs is the most effective way to reduce crime, Marie and Vince weren't quite there yet.

Similarly, Dr. Robert DuPont, a friend of Marie and Vince who worked as a physician in the DC Department of Corrections, noticed that many of the incarcerated men had a history of heroin use. Assuming that heroin led to crime, he started to offer methadone in the jail as a form of rehabilitation. Even today, DuPont's initiative would be considered advanced. Although it is hard to find accurate data on this topic, most carceral facilities do not offer MOUD, and, if they do, its access is extremely limited.[22] Given that at least two-thirds of the country's 2.3 million incarcerated people are estimated to have a substance use disorder, this seems like a significant omission.[23] And, without treatment, release from incarceration is extremely high risk: compared to the general population, people are forty times more likely to die of an opioid overdose within two weeks of being released from prison.[24] When Rhode Island started to offer MOUD in all their correctional facilities, the entire state's overdose rate went down by 12 percent.[25]

Dr. DuPont's methadone program was so successful that he soon expanded it across DC as a whole. By 1970, twenty public methadone clinics were up and running, and, by 1972, the rates of both crime and heroin overdose had dropped.[26] DuPont said that by 1973, they couldn't even find users to enroll in treatment. "It was an experiment that worked, and it worked to a very high level, way beyond anything anyone could have imagined."[27]

Seeing these results, the Nixon administration decided it was time to expand methadone across the entire country. Compared to the expensive social programs that the Democrats wanted, methadone was a cheap way to reduce crime and treat addiction. It also portrayed addiction as a medical disease suffered by individuals, not the systemic problem rooted in societal inequity that it also was.

Moreover, methadone was good for optics: instead of pushing for the incarceration of addicts, Republicans would now be the party pushing for medical treatment.

But Jeffrey Donfeld, one of Nixon's drug policy advisers, knew that methadone maintenance also had to be endorsed by medical experts. Otherwise, it would be written off as just another outlandish idea cooked up by "rightwing wingnuts."[28] So, he reached out to one of the physicians he had met while touring addiction facilities around the country: Dr. Jaffe.

Dr. Jerome Jaffe was a wry, liberal psychiatrist who ran Illinois's Drug Abuse Program. Like every other rising leader in addiction medicine, he had ties to Marie and Vince, having spent six months working in their Rockefeller lab. Dr. Jaffe had a downsloping nose and dark brown eyes encased in large wire-rimmed glasses, and when we spoke on the phone, his dry, outspoken attitude initially felt a little gruff. When he realized that I was a physician, he told me, "If I had known you weren't an aspiring historian, I probably wouldn't have given you the time of day." When I cited some details about his career that I found in a book written by a journalist, Jaffe responded, "The less that is said about that book, the better. When you slant things enough, you can submerge the facts. He's not a historian; he's just trying to make a story. Then he'll go on to something else, like trash in the Pacific or something." I liked Jaffe already.

In 1970, the White House asked Dr. Jaffe to assemble a team of experts to draft a national addiction strategy.[29] His resulting report had several recommendations, including evaluating treatment programs and coordinating a national response, but it was the recommendations around methadone that matter most to this story. By this time, several thousand people had been on methadone for a few years, and there was solid evidence that it was extremely effective.[30] Yet the FDA still considered it an experimental medication, which meant that it was hard to get funding to support methadone programs. As a result, there were an estimated thirty thousand users in the country who had applied for treatment but couldn't get in due to lack of spots.[31] Instead of funding law enforcement, Dr. Jaffe asked for increased funding for treatment. He assumed that this would be a tough sell for the Nixon administration. It wasn't. When Dr. Jaffe briefed Nixon and his cabinet on his recommendations, Nixon agreed to almost every one of them.

Unfortunately, Nixon also resurrected Anslinger's war on drugs. On June 17, 1971, Nixon walked up to a podium emblazoned with the seal of the United States, navy curtains draped behind him, and asked Dr. Jaffe to stand at his side. "Ladies and gentlemen, I would like to summarize a meeting I have just had with the bipartisan leaders." At this point, Nixon leaned in to the podium, pushing his weight into his arms. His brows furrowed. Jaffe stood next to him, clasped his hands, and shifted his gaze from Nixon to the audience in front. Jaffe was young, with long sideburns, a colorful tie, and a suit jacket that was a little too big. Nixon continued, "I began the meeting by making this statement, which I think needs to be made to the nation." He leaned forward even more, so no words would be missed. "America's public enemy number one in the United States is drug abuse. In order to fight and defeat this enemy, it is necessary to wage a new, all-out offensive."[32]

That same day, Nixon signed an executive order creating the Special Action Office for Drug Abuse Prevention (SAODAP), and asked Congress for $371 million to fund it.[33] SAODAP would oversee and fund a vast network of state-run methadone maintenance clinics, and Dr. Jaffe would be in charge as America's first drug czar. Methadone had officially reached its zenith. By 1974, 135,000 patients were in methadone maintenance across the country, and there was very little regulation constraining the way doctors could prescribe it.[34] This was the future that Marie had envisioned for methadone.

It was hard for me to even imagine how exciting this time must have been for Marie. Not only was this what she had been working decades to find—a solution for heroin addiction—but it was spreading quickly across the country and even the world. It felt like a true revolution, one upending decades of criminalization of addiction treatment. I wished I could have been around to feel its momentum.

Methadone's ascension also buoyed Marie. Almost overnight, she went from being viewed as a heretic psychiatrist to one worthy of accolades and fame, with articles about her in *JAMA*, *The New Yorker*, *The New York Times*, and *Vogue*. If she had ever sought confirmation that her approach to addiction was not just some crack-pot idea—which I imagine she had—now there was no question.

When I asked Dr. Jaffe if he found the period exciting, back when he was the country's first drug czar at thirty-seven and methadone was expanding like wildfire, he shared a perspective slightly different than what I predicted. "I guess you could ask somebody in combat whether it was exciting. It's an issue of how you select the words to describe it." He then dove into a monologue about all the battles he constantly had to fight, the uphill battle that was methadone. "So, you ask, was it exciting? It wouldn't be the word I would select."

Whereas I imagine Marie was filled with optimism and hope, Dr. Jaffe had a more realistic view of the challenges ahead, one limited by an expiration date. "I had the feeling, almost from the first day, that the willingness to look at the demand side, rather than the traditional American law enforcement approach, might be a transient phenomenon—that it might pass, and we would go back to our old ways of more and more law enforcement. And I was right. We have never had that proportion of federal resources devoted to intervention on the demand side. We'd never had it before, and we've never had it since. . . . It seemed as if every day was an important day in getting things done, and putting things into place. We really had to move quickly to institutionalize the treatment system so that it would not just decay and fall apart when the current interest in treatment faded."[35]

CHAPTER 11

The Fall

"Would you look at this!" Marie exclaimed as she slapped her fingers across the newspaper. I imagine her and Joyce walking down a crowded Second Avenue, dodging other New Yorkers as they tried to carry on their conversation. It was a humid summer day in 1971, wildflowers and weeds poking up through the cracks in the sidewalk. "Here is another preposterous headline from the medical examiner's office, 'One Person Dying from Methadone Every Hour.'"[1]

Joyce shook her head and furrowed her brow.

"Oh, what a disastrous statement. It's exactly the kind of story that is going to turn everyone against methadone." The tip of Marie's heel tripped over a crack in the pavement as they turned into Stuyvesant Park, but she righted herself without missing a beat.

"Well, that's the point, isn't it?" Joyce asked.

Marie nodded. "I just hate how everybody believes this slander! The medical examiner labels everything as a methadone death. A patient on methadone gets hit by a bus? It's a methadone death! A patient on methadone dies from their advanced cancer? It's a methadone death! It's absolutely tragic, these political games."

"It's all Judy's doing," added Joyce. Judy, or Dr. Judianne Densen-Gerber, was the founder of Odyssey House, one of New York City's most influential therapeutic communities. Ever since methadone received such a large chunk of New York's addiction funding, it seemed she was playing dirty. She reportedly thought the therapeutic communities should have gotten more of the money. Her husband was NYC's deputy medical examiner,[2] and though it can't be proven as intentional, the number of causes of death attributed to methadone increased during this time.[3] Unfortunately, these numbers would later be used as justification by the Bureau of Narcotics and Dangerous Drugs to regulate methadone. It was cited that the percentage of drug-related deaths attributed to methadone by medical examiners increased from 6 percent to 25 percent in New York City from 1970 to 1972.[4]

Just as methadone was proliferating across the world, so, too, were its critics. The *Washington Post* ran inflammatory headlines like "Babies Born Addicted to Methadone: Methadone Causes New-Born Addicts," "Methadone Overdose Kills Youth," and "Patient in Methadone Line is Shot Dead."[5] The *New York Times* wasn't much better.

Newspapers ran article after article about neighborhood associations trying to shut down proposed methadone clinics because they did not want *those* kinds of people coming into their communities. Even though white and Black people used drugs at equal rates, the media often portrayed drug users as young Black men. Marie was convinced that it was an upper-class white lady who got a methadone clinic closed on the Upper East Side because she saw a couple of its Black patients waiting outside for a taxi.[6]

During a press conference, Donald Freeman, the chairman of Citizens Against the Use and Abuse of Methadone, claimed, "Methadone will probably increase the addict population tenfold in the next five to ten years, and help to destroy the Black community."[7] A Democratic congressman stood by his side, as progressives believed that Nixon used methadone as an excuse to shortchange any measures that demanded structural reform. Community members instead asked that the money be spent on playgrounds and food cooperatives, social services that would help prevent addiction in the first place. I could see their point.

In response, Dr. DuPont reassured that the clinics would actually lower local addiction and crime, not incite it—people with addiction were already there. But nobody seemed convinced, perhaps because they knew that as long as methadone was linked to the war on drugs and its primary metric of crime reduction, people on methadone would be treated like criminals.[8] And in America, the image of the criminal has never been race-neutral. As Michelle Alexander writes, "Nothing has contributed more to the systematic mass incarceration of people of color in the United Sates than the War on Drugs."[9]

Methadone became so polarized that Dr. DuPont even received death threats. He told me that *The Washington Post* called him up and said they "had it on good information" that someone was trying to assassinate him.[10] But perhaps it was no surprise after how negatively the media portrayed both him and DC's methadone program. One reporter called Dr. DuPont a fraud who was destroying the city, and a Howard College radio station host told him, "You're killing Black young men and we need to kill you."

If Marie ever received death threats, she never talked about it, but she, too, must have felt these escalating tensions around methadone. Both Dr. Jaffe and Charles Winick said that Marie and Vince started to narrow their circle, only surrounding themselves with pro-methadone friends.[11] Nobody else could be trusted; nobody else could understand.

Marie was particularly upset that the Black community had become one of methadone's fiercest opponents. She did not know how to reconcile her decades-long dedication to treating addiction in Harlem with Black nationalists' growing demands for the eradication of methadone. Many leaders in the Black Panthers and the Young Lords saw methadone as an extension of the state and Big Pharma. Because it continued users' physiologic dependence on opioids, was dispensed by state-controlled clinics led by white people, and required patients to comply with a lot of rules to get their daily dose, methadone was seen as the anathema of self-determination. It was just another form of state control over the Black body. Additionally, activists saw methadone as a weapon used to sedate and pacify the Black resistance. In that regard, it was no better than heroin.[12]

With medicine's poor track record in the Black community, why wouldn't they be suspicious? Racism had been baked into American medicine since the very beginning. Dr. Marion Sims, often credited as the "father of modern gynecology," performed experimental surgeries on enslaved Black women without anesthesia.[13] In 1876, he was named president of the American Medical Association, the largest professional medical society today. In the twentieth century, the AMA persistently supported racial segregation in healthcare.[14] Similarly, it was under the auspices of the federal government that the Tuskegee Syphilis Study occurred. Still, today, Black and Brown Americans tend to receive less and worse care than whites and thus have worse health outcomes.[15]

Surely Marie understood this, herself complaining frequently about the ways in which racism affected the lives of her patients. Yet she did little to try to build their trust. Instead of working with Dr. Beny Primm, a prominent Black addiction physician who directed Brooklyn's methadone program and sought to make it more culturally relevant, she and Vince challenged him simply because he didn't follow their protocols.[16] According to Dr. Primm, Vince and Marie "were adamant that everything be controlled by them and done their way."[17]

Then, along with the critics, came the regulation. First there was the 1970 passage of the Controlled Substances Act, which decreed that scheduling drugs would no longer fall to health officials and the surgeon general, but to the attorney general. Law enforcement would decide how stringently medications such as methadone and, later, buprenorphine would be regulated. Marie and Vince didn't understand why this had been wrested from healthcare's purview; didn't doctors understand medications better than law enforcement? But in a drug war that saw users as criminals and focused on reducing the supply, this change in oversight made sense. Then there was a 1971 FDA ruling that imposed more requirements for methadone yet still maintained its experimental status, refusing to recognize methadone's effectiveness and thereby constraining its use.

Yet the Bureau of Narcotics and Dangerous Drugs still wanted more. In a series of congressional hearings about methadone, the bureau tried to paint a picture of extreme danger: diversion, new addicts, and fatal overdoses. They cited a study in which 87 percent of interviewed heroin users in NYC claimed that someone had tried to sell them illicit methadone at least once in the last six months.[18] They also provided data from undercover police operations

suggesting that physicians were inappropriately prescribing methadone and thus contributing to the black-market supply and leading
opioid-naive citizens to fall under addiction's spell. And, of course,
they mentioned the increasing number of methadone-related deaths
in NYC, a number likely exaggerated by the medical examiner
friendly with therapeutic communities.

Although methadone diversion does exist, medical studies dat-
ing back to the 1970s show that it is not particularly common nor
dangerous. Most diverted methadone is bought by patients who
receive too low of a dose from their clinic or are unwilling or unable to enter formal treatment, and most use it correctly as a form
of self-medication.[19] In a 1995 report, the Institute of Medicine
declared that diverted methadone did not seem to play a significant
role in drug-related deaths, especially when compared to heroin,
and that few people became primarily addicted to methadone.[20] It
was not a major drug of abuse, nor was it particularly hazardous.
There was a small blip in the early 1970s when more heroin users
were misusing methadone because there was a heroin shortage, but
currently, there is no shortage of opioids to get high with.[21] With
a seemingly endless supply of cheap fentanyl, nobody is trying
to get high with methadone or buprenorphine. But if we did want
to reduce MOUD diversion, the most effective approach would be to
increase legal access.[22]

During the COVID-19 pandemic, federal guidelines were loosened so that patients could get four weeks of methadone take-home
doses much sooner, meaning they only had to go to the clinic about
once a month. Over 90 percent of patients said this increased flexi-
bility increased their quality of life;[23] the majority of staff thought
it worked well,[24] and there was no increase in methadone-involved
overdose fatalities.[25] In fact, one study even showed that the number of methadone-involved deaths decreased from 2019 to 2021.[26]
Although SAMHSA's 2024 Final Rule made these pandemic flex-
ibilities permanent,[27] many states and clinics have chosen not to
implement them.[28]

But let's get back to the 1970s. As the congressional hearings
drew to a close, the bureau placed the blame on two main culprits:
script doctors and unscrupulous patients, the same parties targeted

during our country's first drug epidemic. Regulation sought to constrain them both.

As the country's drug czar, Dr. Jaffe found himself in the middle of an increasingly heated debate. When I asked for his side of the story, he replied, "Vince and Marie believed that methadone should be unregulated entirely and left in the hands of the physicians. I didn't agree." Although Marie and Vince didn't need anyone telling them how to practice, they were "a cut above the average general practitioner."[29] Creating regulation was a balancing act: too much and you would restrict access, too little and there would be no quality control.

Additionally, Dr. Jaffe thought increased regulation was needed from a political standpoint. "An accidental overdose is a tragedy," he said, "but you can skip over it when addicts share with each other. But inevitably, you'll have an eight- or six-year-old take the methadone and you'll make headlines." Then even harsher regulations would be created, ones that might completely obliterate any chance for methadone. "Are you willing to risk overdoses of the nontolerant, nonaddicts, and the entire opportunity to treat those who could benefit with that drug? The issue is, you find a way to regulate it, or you will inevitably have these things happen."

I responded: "Of course nobody wants to see a child overdose from methadone, but the reality is they are already dying from accidentally swallowing fentanyl. We had a case like that a few months ago at our hospital." If treatment had been more accessible, perhaps that death could have been prevented.

Nonetheless, I could see Dr. Jaffe's rationale; at the time, diversion was a hot-button issue. Rather than diversion itself being the main problem, it was the handful of high-profile deaths that it would lead to, which would then cause thousands of Americans to lose their access to methadone treatment altogether. As liberals, Black activists, abstinence-based treatment providers, and NIMBY community groups all hated methadone, any death attributable to its misuse was akin to political suicide.

For the first time, someone had convinced me that there was a logical rationale behind today's onerous methadone regulation. I wondered how many of my other hard-line positions should also soften to allow more nuance and empathy. So many times, I had written off physicians who disagreed with me instead of trying to understand their perspective, assuming they were coming from a place of ignorant stigma and didn't have the patient's best interest in mind. But maybe that wasn't the whole story. Maybe it wasn't so black and white. They, too, thought they were doing the right thing.

Although Marie and Vince thought Dr. Jaffe's proposed regulations too stringent, Dr. Jaffe told me they were "not half as tough as they might have been," largely thanks to his pushback. In December 1972, the first version of today's methadone regulations was passed as a series of FDA regulations in Title 21, Code of Federal Regulations, Part 130.[30] In 1973, these regulations were expanded in the form of the Methadone Diversion Control Act and, in 1974, the Narcotic Addict Treatment Act. The latter gave the newly created Drug Enforcement Agency—not Health and Human Services—the authority over the storage and security of drugs used in addiction treatment, including methadone and later buprenorphine.[31] And because these rules were now legislated instead of simply codified by FDA regulations, they were much harder to revise.

Thus, very little about federal methadone regulation has changed since then: Methadone can only be dispensed out of federally recognized methadone clinics, patients can only be enrolled in one program, and there are strict timetables and criteria for granting (and rescinding) take-home doses. The authors didn't expect these stipulations to remain the lay of the land for time immemorial. Rather, they thought the regulations would be loosened as knowledge expanded and methadone maintenance became less controversial.[32] But that day never came, not really. Although they have been slightly modified throughout the years, they haven't changed enough to make a substantial difference. Their most recent amalgamation now lives as Title 42, Code of Federal Regulations, Part 8 (42 C.F.R. § 8).

Although Jaffe's original intent behind these rules was to keep methadone maintenance alive, their impact today is quite the opposite. In 1992, Vince wrote an article blaming increased regulations for the high patient attrition rate in addiction medicine.[33] I, too, blame cumbersome regulations, right up there with stigma and historical precedent, as the reason why it is so hard for patients to access treatment. Why half the country doesn't have access to a methadone clinic. Why less than 2 percent of physicians prescribe buprenorphine and even less methadone. I agree with Marie when she said, "The rules and regulations are to keep people out of treatment."[34]

Despite the short length of 42 C.F.R. § 8, it is not an easy read due to its confusing legal jargon. As a testament to its inaccessibility, SAMHSA, the federal organization charged with overseeing the enforcement of these regulations, has written an eighty-two-page booklet to help explain them.[35] Scared off by such legalese, most doctors I know write off the possibility of giving methadone or buprenorphine to their patients. It is intimidating to offer a medication that comes with almost one hundred pages of legal instructions that might get you in trouble with the DEA if not followed. This isn't a threat that most doctors want to mess around with. Expensive legal fees? A protracted battle with government bureaucracy? The threat of losing one's DEA license? Without a DEA license, no emergency department would hire me. One doctor told me, "If they wanted us to give MOUD, they would say it more clearly." But, of course, the DEA didn't want us to; that was exactly the problem.

The woman sitting across from me on the methadone clinic's gray vinyl couch wore a T-shirt with several horses galloping across her chest, her brown hair in a loose ponytail. Her eyes sagged with creases around the edges, looking much like mine after a late shift in the ED or a morning after the baby had cried all night. On my schedule, she was classified as a "methadone restart," the designation applied when a patient missed at least three consecutive days of coming to get their methadone.

When a patient missed that many days, their dose was knocked back down to 30 milligrams or less, and they had to see a doctor or nurse practitioner to slowly start titrating their dose back up to an amount that would actually prevent craving and withdrawal symptoms, somewhere around 80–120 milligrams. Part of this was federal regulation, part of it was our clinic's interpretation of the rules. We were not supposed to increase the dose any faster than

10 milligrams a day, and, out of an abundance of caution, some providers went even slower. The majority of methadone overdoses occurred during the first week of treatment, when patients adjusted to varying levels of opioids swimming in their bloodstream.

My patients hated such slow titrations, as the medication barely worked at such a low dose. To cope, they often supplemented with fentanyl or heroin. Obviously, this was not ideal—my patients were there because they wanted to stop using. Additionally, the combined use increased the risk of fatal overdose. But, from the doctors' perspective, an overdose from illicit fentanyl couldn't be attributed to their medical care—they hadn't prescribed the street drugs, after all. They had even advised against them! But if a patient overdosed on their prescribed methadone, agents might come knocking.

"Are we almost done?" the woman with the horse shirt asked. Even though she had just arrived in my office, she had already been in the clinic for several hours. Restarts required speaking with a recovery coach and a nurse, repeating urine drug screens, a physical exam, and sitting for another EKG.

"This won't take long," I promised, clicking away at the many boxes in my charting system. I paused to look at her before asking the requisite question: "Why did you miss a few days?" I hated asking this; why was it any of my business why they couldn't make it to the clinic? My doctors didn't know when I missed my prenatal vitamins, but if they did, I doubt they would ask why. At the methadone clinic, however, this was a question we were supposed to ask. And, to be fair, it did have some merit. If they missed because they needed a ride, our recovery coaches could help them. If they missed because they were using, we could discuss increasing their methadone dose.

She sighed, wisps of hair escaping from her hair tie. "I had a family emergency," she began, "and I had to be there. They live out in Jerome." An old mining settlement, Jerome could hardly be considered a town. It was basically just one long street switchbacking over itself as it curved up a steep side of a rocky mountain. There was no methadone clinic for her to "guest dose." And even if there were, it would require a few days to arrange, not something that could be done in the time frame of an emergency. During the COVID pandemic, some clinics even refused to offer such arrangements. One of my patients had to come home early from a family vacation in Hawaii because his guest dosing fell through.

"And so here I am," she continued, "craving something terrible. I couldn't sleep last night because I felt so bad, with nausea and diarrhea and body aches."

We were lucky that she hadn't relapsed, that she came back to us instead of just going on the street. I wished I could have given her a few days' worth of methadone, but she hadn't been at our clinic long enough to earn those kinds of take-home privileges. I wished I could have sent over a prescription to a pharmacy in Jerome, but even though federal regulations allowed methadone prescriptions for pain control, they did not allow it for addiction treatment.

I sighed; this was not the vision that Marie had for methadone. When David Courtwright asked what the future should look like, she answered, "I'd like to see methadone being delivered in every kind of clinic, hospital, and medical plan."[36] Instead of limiting methadone to federally recognized methadone clinics, she wanted any physician to be able to prescribe methadone from any setting: obstetrics, surgery, medicine.

Referring to one of her stable patients, she said, "It's just absurd for them to be stuck in a [methadone] clinic. They don't want to be. They could afford to see a doctor once a month, have a prescription written, go to a drug store, pick it up and have no problem. I think that really is the work we should be doing. I've had patients for seventeen years; they're better rehabilitated than you and I. There has been no drug use for seventeen years and there is no reason in the world why they couldn't have a month's supply, six months' supply, it doesn't matter. If they ever developed a problem, they'd go back into a clinic. There's just no reason. Many of my patients get four months or four weeks' medication; they travel, no problem. There's never been a problem in seventeen years. So I do think that is the future. It's absurd to keep them [in the clinics]. It's part of keeping them isolated and keeping the finger pointed on them and reminding them of what unreliable people they are that they have to be separated into methadone clinics."

Courtwright responded, "Would you require any special training of these physicians? Or is this something you would allow any physician to do?"

Marie emphatically answered, "Oh, I think any physician could do it."

When I first heard Marie's vision for methadone, I almost jumped with excitement. As a relatively new addiction doc starting to see all the barriers standing in patients' way, I knew something needed to change, but I wasn't sure what or how. Just like Marie had trouble envisioning a world where the navy accommodated women, I couldn't imagine a world in which methadone was more accessible. This was before I had joined the advocacy committee of the American Society of Addiction Medicine, before the Modernizing Opioid Treatment Act was proposed, before I completed all the research for this book and became a founding board member of a harm reduction nonprofit, so I was still grasping in the dark. What would an ideal national addiction policy look like? Now here it was, coming directly from the mother of methadone herself. My gut instinct had been right: methadone could be much, much easier to access.

She added: "I think that the prejudices against drug addiction have been going for two thousand years and will continue. Hopefully it will disappear with methadone treatment, with the fact that it is now a medical illness, but it's going to be a long time."

I chuckled at her optimism. Fifty years had passed since our careers and yet, very little had changed. Even if new regulation allows physicians to send methadone prescriptions directly to a pharmacy, barriers will still exist.[37] Just look at buprenorphine. Although any doctor with a DEA license can now prescribe it, most don't, and, even if they did, pharmacists often refuse to fill the prescription. In Appalachia, a region hard hit by the opioid epidemic, one-quarter of pharmacies surveyed in 2016 did not stock bupe, and others admitted to rationing bupe and refusing to fill prescriptions.[38] In a 2021 survey, half of pharmacists cited concerns of a DEA investigation if they filled too many prescriptions or didn't enact enough diversion-prevention policies.[39] Until we radically change our perspectives around demand versus supply, around disease versus crime, around recognizing our shared humanity versus vilifying "the other," nothing will change.

———

Policy and funding, or a lack thereof, would also play a major role in methadone's downfall. As crime rates plummeted, Nixon had less of a political incentive to support methadone. Its job was done. In 1972, Nixon told Congress they were turning a corner in the heroin epidemic.[40] Instead of continuing to lean heavily on the treatment side of drug policy, Nixon began to focus on reducing the supply through enforcement. When he supported mandatory minimums for drug offenses, Dr. Jaffe resigned from his position as drug czar in 1973.

Nixon now had more pressing priorities. As Dr. Jaffe put it, there was "this little thing called Vietnam, this little thing called Watergate."[41] And, so, the funding for addiction treatment began to dry up. In 1974, Nixon introduced an austerity program and SAODAP, along with its multimillion-dollar budget, was dissolved shortly thereafter.

Although Nixon had certainly followed Anslinger's playbook, it was Ronald Reagan who catapulted the war on drugs to the next level. Under Reagan, the funding allocated to federal law enforcement agents to reduce supply soared to quantities I can't even conceptualize—billions of dollars—whereas the funding for addiction prevention and treatment was slashed. SAODAP's successor, the National Institute on Drug Abuse, had its budget reduced from $274 million in 1981 to $57 million in 1984.[42] Although much of that federal funding was reallocated to state authorities via Alcohol, Drug Abuse, and Mental Health Services Block Grants, there was still an overall reduction in treatment capacity.[43] Just as Dr. Jaffe had predicted, the years during which our country prioritized treatment were short-lived.

To justify his war, Reagan sensationalized Black crack-cocaine users. In 1986, the House passed legislation allowing the death penalty for some drug-related crimes and for military participation in narcotics control. The Anti-Drug Abuse Act of 1986 notoriously set mandatory minimums that were one hundred times greater for crack cocaine, associated with Black users, than for powder cocaine, associated with white users.[44] A mere five grams of crack cocaine, an amount that could be consumed during a single binge, meant a mandatory five-year sentence,[45] even for first-time offenders.

It wasn't just Reagan who supported these harsh penalties, but Congress as a whole. The legislation passed 346 to 11, with the majority of dissenting votes coming from the Congressional Black Caucus.[46] Even Democrats advocated for these stringent measures. They didn't want to be known as the party who was soft on crime or drugs, and they wanted to win over white swing voters. Progressives concerned about racial justice largely stayed quiet about the war on drugs, as people with addiction were not a population that most Americans cared about.[47] Instead, the progressives focused on affirmative action as their cause d'être around civil rights. Similarly, few Black leaders saw the war on drugs as a civil rights issue. Instead, they tried to separate themselves as much as possible from the topic, as they already faced enough racism without the added stigma of drug use.[48]

To further punish drug users, the Anti-Drug Abuse Act of 1988 authorized public housing authorities to evict anyone who allowed any drug use to occur—meaning a middle-aged mother might be evicted if her twenty-something-year-old kid smoked some weed while visiting—and eliminated federal benefits, such as student loans, for anyone convicted of a drug offense.[49]

Enforcement became the primary way to fight the war on drugs, with over one million arrests for simple drug possession each year.[50] This figure is six times the number of arrests for the arguably more concerning offenses of drug manufacture or sales.[51] Even after Reagan, this approach persisted. During Bill Clinton's presidency, the incarcerated population grew more than under any other administration.[52] Throughout the entire world, one out of every five people behind bars lives in the United States.[53]

Marie would never live to see most of this. She died in April of 1986 at the age of sixty-seven, her body riddled with cancer. She had been a lifetime smoker. Although she devoted her life to saving others from their addictions, she could not save herself from her own. Her final days were marked by pain as bulbous tumors pressed against nerves and sprouted out of bones.[54] I imagine her lying in bed with Franz Schubert's chamber music echoing softly off the walls and Vince sitting at her side, his hand resting upon hers.

After Marie's death, six months passed before her funeral, perhaps because Vince could not bear to bring himself to see the light of day. According to their friend Paul Brodeur, he sequestered himself within their apartment for that entire time, keeping the drapes drawn. The world outside needed to feel as dark as his heart. The love of his life was gone.

In Courtwright's box of files, I found the program for Marie's memorial. As most of the characters of this book attended, I hoped to find the recording and watch it myself. For over a year, I had been viewing Marie through their books, articles, and interviews, and I longed to see how they moved their hands or shifted their weight when speaking, to hear how their voices broke when heartache burst through their defenses.

Initially, a library archivist told me the tape was lost. The last time it had been viewed was over twenty years ago, and it was impossible to predict where it might have landed. I gave up. But a couple of years later, the recording appeared in my inbox; a journalist had found the tape, digitized it, and passed it to me.

Dr. Robert Newman opened the service with a quote by Marie's mom, Dr. Dorothy Nyswander: "The review of my own work as a health educator has been a painful process. I do not like what I see. It appears to me that most of my efforts were expended in working on the symptoms; the basic conditions giving rise to the symptoms were untouched. Have I not actually helped to maintain the status quo in these situations? Have I not taught people to accept those gifts approved by the establishment, which would make life more bearable but which would not threaten the power of establishment itself? Deep down I have dreams that you, my students, will not repeat my sins of omission, that you will do better."

Hearing some of my deepest concerns reflected, tears formed. Of course, I did not believe that Dorothy was referring to methadone as the symptomatic treatment, but to the ways in which the medical establishment tended to co-opt and whitewash practices rooted in self-determination and social justice. For example, taking over methadone maintenance and turning it into a system of control and enforcement, forcing people to take methadone via mandatory treatment or face jail time. Or taking over naloxone distribution in a way that ignored its grassroots origins and discarded the radical tenets of harm reduction. Did the house always have to win? And if Dorothy and Marie hadn't figured out the answer to that question, how could I?

Then Dr. Beatrice Berle stood up, reminiscing about working together at their Harlem clinic before closing with a prescient line about Marie's legacy: "We are still, and always will remain, under the influence of Marie, a great human being. Straightforward, loving, but not sentimental, objective, not judgmental, breathing life and health with her presence and a few words, her influence persists, will be with us, within us, all our lives. That is Marie Nyswander's immortality which we share."

Dr. Mary Jeanne Kreek spoke next, referring to Marie as her mentor and recounting the thrill of success during methadone's early days. Yet, despite her achievements, Marie never became complacent, always moving the goalpost forward. When adolescents were excluded from the city's first methadone maintenance programs, she started one that would treat them. In the 1980s, "she resisted the regulations and over-restrictiveness which kept successful patients from being able to accept continued treatment." When she wasn't working, Marie turned to nature, whether at her Connecticut cottage or in the wide-open spaces of the West, and "she wanted to assure that same freedom for all." In closing, Dr. Kreek said we can continue to recognize Marie's presence "in the joyous spirit of each person" successfully treated with methadone.

Subsequent friends and colleagues came to the podium, some of whom I recognized, some who were new, but all remembered her humor, unrivaled rapport with patients, free spirit, love of travel, and boundless enthusiasm for life.

The ceremony closed with Vince, who stood from the front row wearing what appeared to be a white rose on his lapel. He spoke for less than two minutes, perhaps still too bereft for a polished soliloquy: "To live a full life is not a small thing."

Through her work, Marie had found a way to live beyond her corporeal form, traces of her radiating outward into the world via her friends and colleagues. Her impact on addiction medicine would be passed on from teacher to trainee, over and over again, even if they didn't know her name. And, maybe, even to me.

CHAPTER 12

Unanswered Questions

2021

It was a Friday morning when Paul Brodeur and I first spoke.[1] Among Courtwright's papers, Brodeur was mentioned as someone who knew Marie and Vince, and, unlike many of their acquaintances, he was still alive. Not knowing anything else about him, I sent a message through his website, and he wrote back almost instantly. "Yes," he responded, "I was a close friend of Marie, Vince, and Leonard. I would be glad to chat with you about them."

We talked for almost two hours, his enthusiasm spilling through the phone as my fingers flew across the keyboard to catch every word. Although I did not know it at the time, he was a successful environmental journalist who doggedly exposed the hazardous effects of asbestos and chlorofluorocarbons. His 1968 *New Yorker* article is sometimes compared to Upton Sinclair's novel *The Jungle* in its significance, as it caused such a stir that Congress mandated asbestos's removal from schools.[2] When we spoke, he was likely calling from his modernist home in Cape Cod, a collection of cement hexagons piled in the woods.[3] According to his daughter, he fished and gardened so much during retirement that he was practically self-sustaining.[4]

I began our conversation by asking, "How did you meet Marie?"

"I met Marie when she was married to Leonard, back in 1958."

Leonard was Marie's third husband, the one she divorced to marry Vince. A lay psychiatrist, he needed a physician to sign off on his charts, prescribe medications, and go over cases.[5] That's how he met Marie.

Brodeur continued: "He was the uncle of my best friend and worked at *The New Yorker*, so, when the magazine offered me a job, I asked him what I should do. He said, 'Don't be crazy! That's a literary stipend for life!'" Brodeur took his advice. "That started my long mentorship that lasted as long as Lenny lived. He was my older brother and mentor, and I loved him the way I have never loved anybody outside my own family."

Brodeur then shifted to Marie. "She was a sportswoman, sort of rugged. She had grown up out in Utah and had done a lot of camping. Dorothy bought Marie and Leonard twelve acres of land with a tiny cottage with no plumbing in Newtown, Connecticut. Leonard was not an outdoor guy at all, not even a smidgen, and he and Marie tried to live there. You had to bring water in from a siphon up the hill. Can't see another house."

Eventually, they gave up, bought a real house, and told Brodeur he could have the cabin. At the time, it was so shabby that trees were growing through the windows, but Brodeur turned it into a writing studio that somehow felt in the middle of nowhere despite being only an hour from New York City.

When Marie fell in love with Vince, Leonard tried to win her back by building her a cabin at the top of a hill only three hundred yards from Brodeur's Connecticut home. Although his scheme didn't work, Marie made good use of the cabin. Brodeur said, "Marie and Vince came to the cabin every weekend, and every Saturday night they came over to my house and cooked a London broil on the Franklin stove. Vince became sort of a grandfather to my children and Marie was like a big sister to me. She was a wonderful woman. I adored her." For twenty years they continued this tradition. At Vince's seventieth birthday party, Brodeur jovially recounted the story of his young son's first solo journey at age two, a hike up the hill and through the woods to their cabin.

As Brodeur wove through the dramas of their lives, it felt as if I was sitting upon a rug in their cottage, a fire in the hearth, a cup of cider in my hands. After he told me about Leonard and Vince's love lives after Marie, we circled back to the topic at hand—methadone. And that's when he dropped the bomb: "[Vince], of course, was the lead guy on methadone. He had discovered that it was a heroin block."

Here it was again, the same suspicion voiced by the *Addiction* editor in his letter to Courtwright. "I have sometimes been left wondering whether Nyswander was in truth more important to Dole as a person than as a scientific collaborator."

How could anyone believe such a thing? Marie was a leading addiction physician with decades of experience, a published book, and a track record of pushing against the status quo time and time again. At Narco, she was one of the first physicians in the world to give methadone, and she had supported the idea of opioid maintenance therapy long before it was a thing. The better question might be, how could methadone maintenance not have been her idea? Was it simply that the editor could not fathom a world in which such innovation came from a woman? When would her accolades ever be enough?

In my professional life, I often feel that if I just have more certifications and papers and titles, then people will listen to me. I'm not the only one; according to studies, many female physicians share this tendency. Recently, I tried to explain to a provider that it was safe to let our postpartum patient taking buprenorphine breastfeed, even citing evidence, but she refused to listen, instead telling me this was all just my opinion. I wanted to scream and cry hot tears of frustration, mainly for this mom and her baby, but also for me. Even as the director of our hospital's addiction medicine consult service, a position I accepted in 2022, I still didn't have enough legitimacy. But if all the accomplishments in the world still weren't enough for Marie, I didn't stand a chance.

In this world where the accomplishments of women and people of color have historically been omitted, it felt important to both get Marie's individual history right and to correct a false historical record at large. There is power in history; otherwise, politicians wouldn't be trying so hard to ban the books that tell it.[6] Until Marie receives the credit she is due, the omission is not just an injustice isolated to the past but still ongoing, still obstructing our path forward. For my daughters to envision careers as leaders and scientists, they need to see examples that look like them.

"You don't think it was Marie?" I asked Paul.

"No," he answered firmly. "I never ever, ever got that impression from either one of them. I always had the impression that it was Vincent. This is from news accounts, from conversations with both of them, etcetera. I do not think that was possible."

"Do you think it was possible that it was Marie's idea, but she wanted to promote Vince?" I asked. Perhaps, during that time in history, it was not socially acceptable to be as successful as your husband. Perhaps she was trying to be the good wife.

Paul considered before answering. "I don't think Marie was that self-effacing. She was a modest woman, but I think it's very unlikely that either one of them would let him take credit if it wasn't his. He was a very honest, honorable man. I don't think he would have deprived his own wife of credit that she deserved. That doesn't go over with anything I know about Vincent Dole." Then the tone in Paul's voice shifted, a lightheartedness finding its way in. "This is a long time ago! It's going to be difficult for you, since everyone they know has died."

I nodded. Even after all these interviews, all these archival requests, I would never know for sure.

He asked, "Do some people believe that Marie thought of it?"

"Yes," I answered. "Dr. Joyce Lowinson, a physician who worked closely with her at Rockefeller, unwaveringly credits Marie."

Joyce took my call from her apartment study at the Lombardy, an elegant Manhattan building built in the 1920s.[7] As we spoke, I imagined her on a green fainting couch placed alongside built-in bookshelves that reached the ceiling.

When I asked if she thought methadone might have been Vince's idea, she was so shocked by the suggestion that she took a few seconds to respond.

When she finally spoke, there was not a trace of hesitation in her voice. "The idea of methadone for heroin addiction was *her* idea. Not his."

Relief coursed through my body, and I let out a loud sigh.

Joyce told a version of a story I had heard before, but, this time, attribution was assigned. "They had two heroin addicts who were admitted to the hospital and Dole was treating them with morphine. These two guys were up at the nurses' station every couple of hours asking for their next dose. And Marie suggested that they try methadone, as it was longer acting. She had used it in a detox capacity at Lexington. It worked so quickly, that after a couple of days, these guys were up there asking how to help the nurses!"

Out of everyone I had spoken to, Joyce was the only one who had worked alongside Marie at Rockefeller, the only one who had been there before, during, and after methadone's discovery. She was also the only other woman I spoke with, as well as Marie's best friend. She was even her bridesmaid when Marie and Vince married. Out of everyone, I trusted her account the most.

And, of course, there had been Courtwright's written response to the *Addiction* editor, typed onto a thin piece of paper and filed within the cardboard box he mailed me:

"In answer to your question as to the exact role Marie Nyswander played in the Dole–Nyswander collaboration, I would say that she was rather more than a full partner in spotting and understanding the potential significance of the early methadone maintenance trials. . . . Was she more important to Dole as a person than as a scientific collaborator? That's a shrewd question. There's no question that she reenergized his life. Yet I'd have to answer in the negative. Without her savvy, insight, and rapport with patients, I don't think Dole would have gotten as far with methadone maintenance, at least not in the early stages. He might even have dropped the project. Historians call this 'counterfactual speculation,' and while I'm certainly happy to share my thoughts with you in a letter, I wouldn't care to open that particular can of worms in the article. Putting Nyswander posthumously on the couch is likely to be controversial enough."

Pride coursing through me, I sat a little taller in my seat. Together, it felt like we were backing up a good friend, supporting her legacy when others tried to tear it down. His words made me trust both his perspective—he seemed to be a true ally who was handling her story with care—and my own. From the clues and fragments of her life, I had correctly assembled the puzzle.

Yet a question continued to plague me. Why would Marie act like methadone was all Vince's creation if it weren't true? Perhaps she was just trying to be the ideal wife, the one she profiled in her first book, *The Power of Sexual Surrender*.[8]

In 1959, three years after she published *The Drug Addict as a Patient* and while she was working with Dr. Beatrice Berle in East Harlem, Marie published another kind of book, *The Power of Sexual Surrender*. The book was the result of the problems she saw while working as a marital therapist, an area of psychiatry that perhaps she would have pursued more if addiction had not co-opted her career. Many women came to her for advice about sex and relationships, and Marie blamed the modern feminist movement for causing their "frigidity."

In the book, she painted a picture of how the ideal woman behaved. For starters, "she is very, very glad to be a woman, with all the duties, responsibilities, and joy it entails. She can't imagine what it would be like to be a man and has no interest in imagining it as a possible role for herself. She feels that the very existence of her husband makes the world safe for her." I wanted to vomit—did Marie really believe this crap? Marie then described how the ideal woman was biologically predestined to give the best of herself to her husband, this disposition bringing her joy and balance in life. She also "believes firmly in the fact that marriage is a sacrament, binding forever," yet another statement that was quite contrary to how Marie lived her own life.[9]

The book then gets even weirder, delving into the sex life of the ideal woman. "She's not very modest, I'm afraid. In fact, she's quite a show-off and likes sexual compliments from her husband, dressed or undressed, verbal or otherwise. . . . She's not sexually shy at all. She wouldn't demur a moment at initiating love with her husband, though she will immediately change her amorous direction if she finds he is too tired or is preoccupied, without feeling the least bit rejected. . . . She knows this: that it is the man who, from the purely physical viewpoint, has to be ready before sexual intercourse can take place. . . . That is why (by virtue of that deeper sense of reality we spoke of) when her husband is ready to make love our lady is nearly always willing. . . . But she not only takes the lead from him about *whether* they are going to make love—the *kind* of love they are going to make is also usually his decision and, in pure delight, she follows him completely."

Marie wrote that her female clients often complained that this ideal woman was "a victim of the male" and "an impossible ideal." I would have to agree.

When I first stumbled across this book, I didn't know where to place it within the scope of her life. Of course, I wanted to see the version of Marie that was a feminist success story. In addition to becoming a physician when few women did, she also assembled a team of women who went on to become leaders in their own right: Dr. Beatrice Berle, Dr. Joyce Lowinson, Dr. Francis Gearing, and Dr. Mary Jeanne Kreek. Although representation wasn't enough, it was still worthwhile, each woman having the chance to pull several more up behind her. How did this same person write such a nutty, misogynistic book?

Paul Brodeur laughed when I asked him what he thought about *The Power of Sexual Surrender*. "I don't know. We were always hoping we would meet women like that." Even though Marie was listed as the sole author, Brodeur believed that Leonard wrote most of the book, Marie just supplying the sex scenes. "I don't think either one of them believed it, frankly. It wasn't like Marie at all. I think it was a very hot-selling subject. Lenny had been an editor and a writer, so he probably had an idea that such a book would sell like hotcakes. It was a very titillating book, and they probably made some money on it, which is maybe why they wrote it."

Yet this book wasn't a one-off. In 1962, Marie was quoted extensively in a newspaper article under the headline "Women ARE Different from Men!" claiming that women and men were biologically different and thus should be educated differently. Ultimately, the woman's place was in the home. She wrote, "There's a crying need for women's colleges to stop turning into men's schools. Instead, some brave school should stand up and say, 'Women are different, have God-given gifts, and let's see where a woman's pleasure does come from—from chemistry 203 or from keeping the love level high in a family!'"[10] Again, her advice rang with a sense of distorted hypocrisy.

When I asked Courtwright if he thought Marie meant what she wrote, he smiled and shrugged his shoulders.[11] He had wondered the same. According to his interview with Charles Winick, the book landed Marie on a feminist shitlist with the second-wave feminist Robin Morgan. This infuriated Marie, as she saw herself as a liberated career woman. How bizarre that she did not see that coming.

For more insight, Courtwright recommended that I review a letter currently held in the University of Montana's archives. After Marie and Leonard divorced, he eventually married a poet who became the love of his life. When they first met, she wrote a letter gushing to a friend about this wonderful man. But also in the letter were some less savory parts of his history that made her a little nervous: "He's 55. He's been married three times: for 12 years very unhappily, then another time, most happily and lengthily, to Marie Nyswander. . . . But all of a sudden she broke it up, upset by fame, a scarring cancer operation, a sudden lover. He was desperately unhappy."[12]

"A scarring cancer operation?" Courtwright repeated back to me. "Now, you're a doctor. In a woman who desperately wanted kids, and who was described as a second mother by many, what does this suggest to you?"

I blinked. "Cervical cancer? A hysterectomy?" I suggested.

Courtwright nodded quietly in response. He had come to the same conclusion. My critiques of Marie's feminism softened. Although mothering and working during a pandemic stretched me thin, there was also an extreme contentment that came with parenthood, one that Marie would never know. Maybe *The Power of Sexual Surrender* was a testament to another life she wanted but could never have.

Courtwright also suggested that Marie's relationship with her parents might have played into her ideas about the sanctity of the home. They separated when Marie was barely a baby, perhaps creating some anxiety about loss and love. Although it did not seem like her dad was involved in her life, Marie idolized her mom. Dorothy's successful public health career obviously influenced Marie's path.

After residency, Marie even worked at the same New York City health department where Dorothy completed her seminal study. When Marie wrote her first book, *The Drug Addict as a Patient*, she dedicated it to her mom.

Yet they were not particularly close. When Marie was a little girl, Dorothy was rarely around. She worked during the day and earned her PhD at night, and it was the babysitter and Dorothy's parents who watched little Marie. After Dorothy became a professor, the long-distance business trips began. Sometimes she spent entire summers out of state. When I asked Joyce Lowinson about their relationship, she told me it "was complicated. She admired her mom, but the relationship was not close. Dorothy was independent." Independent was certainly one word for it; Marie didn't even tell her mom when she enrolled in medical school or got married.[13]

In asserting that women should focus on the sanctity of the home, perhaps Marie was writing from a place of childhood yearning. On the one hand, Marie worshipped her mom and all her successes, while, on the other, she wished she were around more. Both things could be true. I wondered if my own daughters would feel the same conflict about us.

I couldn't figure out how to reconcile Marie's dueling personas. But perhaps I didn't need to. Instead, I could practice radical empathy, a virtue described by writer Steve Almond as one that allows us to hold empathy for people whose views we disagree with, people who are products of competing ideologies.[14] To be clear, this does not mean that we need to subscribe to their beliefs or excuse their actions. Rather, we recognize their humanity and treat them with care. Marie could hold multiple identities and truths at once, even when they conflicted. She was my role model, not the gold standard.

CHAPTER 13

Grassroots

2021

Every day, I checked my email to see if the hospital CEOs had approved the press release about our upgraded addiction services. Weeks passed, and, still, nothing—what could be taking them so long? Our statement had been clear and concise, and it portrayed our hospital in a favorable light: We were leading the way in addiction care and serving our community. It should have been a quick turnaround, but the longer it took, the more people we missed.

Then, one afternoon while working a shift in the emergency department, the response finally arrived. The email did not come from the CEOs themselves, but from the public information officer, and, as I read, all the commotion around me faded into the background: the chatter of the residents, the dance music pulsing from the speakers, the beeping monitor in the hallway. I leaned forward in my swivel seat, hinging at my hips and allowing my large belly to balance on my outstretched thighs—I was now eight months pregnant with my second daughter. Did the last month of pregnancy always have to be stressful?

The public information officer wrote, the CEOs "are happy we are providing the care and enhanced services, but they wonder if this is something the other ED's in town are doing or if our teams are the only ones. If so, does EMS know we are providing this service—will they bring all suspected OD/addiction patients to us because of this service? They are concerned that if we announce this publicly, that we will become the city's primary resource for substance abuse."

Fast rage spat through my fingers and clacked loudly across my keyboard as I replied. So what if we became the city's main resource for substance use? We were the university hospital, offering many services that smaller facilities did not. We were already the region's "main resource" for trauma, transplant, pediatrics, etcetera, and we often boasted about our ability to treat anything. Why was this any different? Additionally, the community relied on us to provide care to the most vulnerable. My response was peppered with phrases like "standard of care," "cost-effective," and "public acclaim." Wasn't that what the C-suite cared about, after all? I even offered to provide research and data to allay their concerns. Surely that would be enough to remove any doubts they might have. I pressed Send. Then a resident appeared at my side, and the din returned to the room. There were patients to see.

Several days passed before their reply arrived. "Hi everyone, our CEOs would prefer not to send out a media announcement on the topic. They would be happy to share the announcement internally in our leadership message. I'll share with our internal communications manager."

My jaw dropped with disbelief. There were often public announcements showcasing our cardiac or stroke care—how was this any different? The difference was they would rather people who used drugs die than seek care at our hospital. Although I doubted they lost any sleep over their decision, I couldn't let it go.

I thought about their email throughout our family dinner and while my daughter splashed in the bathtub. I tried to remain calm as I read bedtime stories from the colorful board books that lined her bedroom shelves, even though indignation simmered under my skin. It wasn't until I reached overhead to turn off her light that I felt even a tinge of relief, because now, finally, I would have time to draft my reply. Instead of burrowing under the blankets, drowsy with dopamine after our snuggles, I padded across the dark house to the office, switched on the light, and began to type as the glowing computer screen illuminated my face.

Whose doors could I bang down? Should we assemble a team to write the state medical director? But what would we ask? Beg her to ask our hospital's CEOs to write a press release? It sounded ridiculous. There was that journalist who wrote about our fire department's naloxone program—maybe I could ask her to do a story that wasn't authorized by our hospital. Would any of the other addiction docs join me? I wrote to the others on my team, asking them to help brainstorm next steps. Although a handful would reply, the conversation would soon die off, quickly neglected for issues seen as more pressing. People who used drugs weren't politically important. Neither was I. There was nothing I could do. I hated feeling so powerless.

As had been true in Marie's day, supporting MOUD was equivalent to fighting an uphill battle. In an interview aired on PBS in 2000, Dr. DuPont surmised, "Methadone was just horrible from a political point of view, just a total disaster. It was an orphan from beginning to end, and it is today. I think the simplest way to say it is that it's an addicting drug. How can you treat addiction with an addicting drug? At the end of the day, you're not going to make that sale. It's not going to happen. So we never got over that problem, and it was always pushing a rock up a mountain, only to have it fall back down on you over and over again."[1] Of course, dependence is different than addiction, so I would not agree with DuPont's categorization of methadone as an addicting drug, but, still, he had a point.

No matter how many studies I presented showing the benefits and safety of MOUD, no matter how many cost-analyses showed that it reduced costs, no matter how many successful policies I showcased—nothing seemed to be enough to change the hearts of those who didn't "believe in" MOUD, as if it were an opinion instead of the evidence-based medical treatment it was. During her career, Dr. Frances Gearing had been equally baffled by her inability to change scientific minds about methadone. If something that should be as undisputed as treatment was so politically disastrous, what did that say about the even more controversial interventions of overdose prevention centers, syringe distribution, and drug decriminalization? I was coming to understand that as stigma did not live in the rational part of our brains, it could not be swayed by facts and figures.

I sighed and stared out the dark window, the Santa Catalina mountains hidden by shadows. I now understood the frustration in Christopher's voice when he had to explain why people who used drugs deserved to live, the deep exhaustion that came from saying the same thing, over and over again, upon deaf ears.

I wished I could turn to Marie. I imagined that she also had felt like Sisyphus, fatiguing herself day after day with the seemingly impossible task of reducing stigma and expanding access to methadone, goals that still felt light-years away. Did she ever let herself fully rest, or was she like me, her mind always racing toward the next step? In the tapes with David Courtwright, she always sounded so cheerful, a jovial tone singing through her words. I longed to call her up and ask her advice: "Marie, when you wanted to give up, when you felt all alone, when with every step forward, regulations or politics took you two steps back—where did you find your fortitude? How did you keep going? And, even more importantly, how did you do it with joy?"

Into my internet browser, I typed a job posting I had recently seen for an addiction position out of state. Scrolling through the description, I coveted their large cadre of faculty to research, teach, and treat patients, as well as support staff to coordinate care and collect data. At my hospital, I was the only addiction attending. Think of what I could accomplish with that kind of support! I imagined myself like Marie, walking up to the stage at a large medical conference to talk about some innovative clinical tool I had developed.

If I stayed at my hospital, I'd never get the resources needed to spearhead something so forward-thinking. I would never develop something as monumental as methadone, because my days would instead be filled with simply trying to attain a basic quality of care for people with chaotic drug use and to convince hospital leadership that their lives mattered. Whereas Marie and her hospitals had been on the front page of *The New York Times*, we couldn't even make it into the local paper, because our hospital tried to hide us in the shadows. I would never become *somebody* like Marie. And, although my initial indignation was too self-centered, it was a smoke signal for the real issue at hand: how little value my hospital placed on addiction medicine and our patients.

Although I had inadvertently broken the law in Michigan when I prescribed buprenorphine, now, I was about to do so deliberately. The copper sun dipped behind the dramatic peaks of the Tucson Mountains, sharp pyramids of granite reaching toward the sky. I was waiting in my car for a man I had never met. Only one other car was in the parking lot, an old gray sedan with its side door swung open sitting at the opposite end of the long stretch of pavement. But that's not to say the park was empty. Small congregations of people scattered across the dry, yellowed grass, and a few were lying by themselves in patches of shade. Most were older, and there were no kids to be seen.

Although the sun's intensity was waning, my car thermometer still said it was 105 degrees. A man biked across the sidewalk with a second bike propped over his front handlebars and a third balanced over his rear rack. A woman leaned against the brick wall of the neglected baseball field, her hiking boots, baggy canvas pants, and long-sleeved denim shirt caked in a layer of dust. Had my presence been similarly noticed?

I was waiting for Joby, a twenty-three-year-old who worked for Sonoran Prevention Works and described himself as "a white-passing, cis male who used heroin and meth chaotically and speedballed every morning."

A car pulled up next to mine, leaving less than a couple of feet between us. I assumed it must be him—who else would park so close when there was so much space? I rolled down my window as the driver stepped out, a young man with short black hair. "Are you Joby?" I asked, my voice wavering.

His eyes darted to his two friends getting out of the car, a woman and a man with a skateboard. "No, no," he said, walking away from me as quickly as possible.

Did he think I was looking to buy drugs? Or meetup with a hookup from Tinder? Probably the latter, as, with the bulky car seat strapped into the backseat, I could pass for a bored mom or housewife. And maybe I was. Why else would I be here, meeting a man that I knew nothing about, to hand out syringes illegally, while my husband was at home reading to our toddler? Not only was I missing her bedtime routine, but I was threatening our entire family's stability. I was about to commit a felony.

I certainly didn't want to get arrested or thrown into jail while pregnant, especially not during the pandemic. Pregnancy meant that I was at greater risk of severe complications from COVID-19, and I knew from working in the ED that death was not outside the realm of possibility. Additionally, like Marie, I knew that an arrest and an open court case would threaten my ability to help patients. While the case dragged on, my hospital and the state medical board would likely forbid me from seeing patients. But I couldn't keep waiting until the CEOs were finally ready—too many lives would be lost.

Warren was uncharacteristically supportive of tonight's civil disobedience and kept texting to ask how it was going. Usually, he was the one who abided by the rules, unable tell a lie to save his life. On some level, we must have both sensed that tonight's "good trouble" offered something important.[2]

Although I had briefly considered leaving Tucson to join a hospital more supportive of addiction, the idea was fleeting. This was where I went to college, where Warren and I bought our first home and planted our first garden. With each passing season, the yard's foliage became lusher: the mesquites reaching up to the telephone lines, globe mallows forming an impenetrable wall along the rain basin, and blackfoot daisies spilling over the planter edge. I had never before lived somewhere long enough to watch my dreams grow into reality. I started to learn my neighbors' stories, to recognize the trill of a gila woodpecker and the song of the curve billed thrasher. Finn was best friends with a girl she met when they were just babies, and I loved watching their games mature with each passing month. For the first time, I had lived somewhere long enough for layers of meaning to imbue everything around me. We couldn't leave now.

Although the hospital might not care about addiction, people in Tucson did. Just like everywhere else in the country, almost everyone knew someone affected by substance use. Addiction was here, whether the hospitals wanted to admit it or not, and I could help. There was work to be done. Wasn't that why I pursued medicine in the first place? To make the world a better place?

Through the windshield, I watched a boxy black Toyota Corolla make a sweeping turn into the lot, looking like it had arrived straight from the nineties. The driver was a wiry man with straight hair reaching his shoulders, angular eyebrows, and scraggly facial hair. He saw me and waved. I turned off the engine, swung my canvas bag over my shoulder, and headed his way.

Joby jumped out of his car, popped the trunk, and started pulling boxes from the stuffed compartment. In doing so, he jostled a jumper cable, its alligator clamp now dangling over the rear bumper. His hair was lazily dyed blond, his dark brown roots long and very much visible, and his eyes were a mix of blue and brown sprinkles. He wore a baggy white T-shirt, loose black shorts, and mismatched socks, one white and one black, both scrunched above his ankles. His left foot was not yet entirely in his shoe, his heel flattening the edge of the black canvas. His forearms and calves were decorated by several tattoos, all looking a little homemade. My eye kept returning to one on his arm, a tombstone with the inscription "Going nowhere fast."

As he rifled through his supplies in some kind of effort to sort them, my body instinctively leaned forward to help. A second passed before I caught myself—I had no idea how things should be organized. It was time for me just to watch and listen.

"These are the syringes," he explained, pulling out several boxes. "We have shorts," which had needles that were five sixteenths of an inch, "and longs," with needles that went up to half an inch. "These are sort of smaller volumes, so they aren't as popular as the one hundred units, but we'll still run out."

I didn't quite understand; how could we run out? There were so many syringes here. But, before I could ask, he had already moved on.

"These are the McKessons, which aren't as desirable, as the needle is duller. It hurts more. But our syringes are either donated or stolen, so." He shrugged. He started to pack everything into two large duffle bags, one for each of us to carry. I wondered where they came from—the hospital? His partner was a nurse, so it seemed possible.

He started to pack tiny packages of soap, pads, tampons, and combs into Ziplock bags. Then he moved to the pipes. "We have meth and crack pipes that we give out. From a distributor in California. About fifty cents a pipe. They break easily, but they are so affordable."

I could see what he meant—both were made of a thin glass and no more than four inches long with a stem less than a centimeter in diameter. The pipe for meth ended in a round sphere, and the pipe for crack was just a thin cylinder with a tiny fabric rose at one end.

"They put the rose in so they can get away with selling them. We leave it in, 'cause, well, they're kind of cute." He held the thin glass tube in his hand, flipping it back and forth. "They put Brillo pads in here."

"Why?"

"To hold the crack in place, I guess. Maybe like a filter. I'm not really sure." He grabbed a handful from the trunk and stuffed them into the duffle. As he reached for more, he asked, "Do you feel comfortable carrying the pipes and syringes? It's illegal." His eyes met mine. "Some people have a record and can't be arrested again, so I want to make sure everyone knows."

"How often do the police mess with you?" I asked. I was wearing a black-and-white shirt with an illustration of a bicycle next to a saguaro under a full moon, cutoff army-green shorts, and soft-soled tennis shoes that were basically slippers. I didn't look that different from the folks in the park.

"Oh, a fair bit. They usually come out to the park once or twice a day, and they harass anyone giving things out."

As we walked the southern border of the park, I watched a van pull up to the other end of the parking lot, swing open their back doors, and extricate a folding table, crates of cold water, and a giant vat of soup. Perhaps it was a church.

Joby continued: "Usually, they tell us that they know we are giving things out, but we deny it, and they tell us to leave. We stuff everything in the trunk and drive off. Then they push everyone else out of the park, out into the washes where they are harder to see." Washes were the dry ditches lined by mesquite trees that crisscrossed all over Tucson, their banks swelling into rivers during the summer monsoons. He shook his head. "Then it's hard for me to find them."

Before tonight, I would have said no, instead focusing my efforts solely within the system. But, after the CEOs' response, I realized that not only had my approach been futile, but I may even have caused harm. In trying to convince leadership that people who used drugs deserved care, I pandered to what I thought they wanted to hear. Instead of sharing the more radical components of harm reduction, I preached only the narrative of redemption: someone hits rock bottom, they decide they want help, and a doctor races in to save them. With the help of medication, they stop using heroin or fentanyl, mend broken relationships, find fulfillment at work, and move off the streets and into a house. It was the same upwardly mobile story we told ourselves about life in America. Work hard enough, and you will be successful. It was what people wanted to hear.

Unfortunately, it wasn't the whole truth. For people with chaotic drug use, their story sometimes lacked a clear plot or thesis. Things did not always happen for a reason. Sometimes the protagonist failed to evolve in any significant way. Many fell sick, lost their families, and became unemployed, yet they continued to use. Instead of resulting in a satisfying ending, the story often fizzled out. For them, my crisp arc of salvation was no more than a fairy tale. Even worse, it suggested that only people who wanted to get sober were deserving of care.

Just as Dorothy had so eloquently cautioned, my actions thus far had only served to support the status quo. Although my hospital now offered naloxone and MOUD, the shame and the punishment still remained, as did the hierarchical approach that placed physicians at the pinnacle. I have watched doctors—many of whom would start MOUD on patients committed to sobriety—refuse to listen to their patients' needs, treat them with scorn, or withhold care and treatment, simply because of their desire to continue to use substances. If we want to actually support our community and turn the tide of our country's overdose epidemic, we need to do more than just pass out naloxone and start MOUD; we need to completely reframe our approach to include all the aspects of harm reduction, not just those that are politically palatable. We have to center users' goals and priorities above our own, even if it makes us uncomfortable.

Time and time again, my mind had changed around addiction: first seeing it as a nuisance, then as a medical condition with treatment, to viewing methadone as a powerful solution that should be much more available, and, now, to seeing harm reduction as a goal worthy in its own right instead of just a bridge to recovery. At any one time, only 5 percent of people with substance use disorder want treatment.[3] Yet, if healthcare providers even talk about addiction, it is usually only that small subset that we focus on. Everything revolves around entering treatment, starting MOUD, and getting "clean." But what about everyone else? By focusing exclusively on treatment, we are effectively turning our backs on anyone who didn't agree with us, saying that we will only help if they truly want to quit. Physicians had simply taken the moral model of Marie's day, cloaked it in a white coat, and renamed it the medical model.

So, here I was, taking my first steps along a new path, still unsure where they might lead. If my hospital system didn't even want to let the community know that we could treat addiction, if they refused to care about the humanity of people who used drugs, I would have to start working outside the system, following the lead of Haley, Christopher, Joby, and all the other brilliant minds I had met through Sonoran Prevention Works.

Additionally, it felt unfair to be out here with Joby without putting any skin in the game. If he were risking his livelihood to help others, then so would I. This was what it meant to be an ally. As Martin Luther King Jr. said, "One has a moral responsibility to disobey unjust laws."

"I understand it's illegal," I told Joby. "I can carry them." I reached my open palms toward the collection of pipes in his grasp, and, without missing a beat, he handed them over.

Joby then moved on to arranging other supplies: alcohol wipes, antiseptic ointment, tiny packets of ibuprofen, tourniquets, clean cotton, and cookers in which to heat and dissolve certain drugs. As this whole process took about fifteen minutes, he apologized for the delay. By this point, we had long been spotted, and people were gradually milling closer. First, a man with his slick black hair woven into two French braids, meticulously parted along the middle, his face completely covered by tattoos. When we asked if he knew how to use the naloxone, he said, "I gave it once to someone who fell out. Just last week someone fell out here." He swept his arm out over the park. As he started to walk away, he turned to ask one last question, "Can you give it in the chest? *Pulp Fiction* style?" He smiled.

We recommended against it.

After giving out kits to the five or so people who had approached, we picked up our duffle bags and weaved through the circles of people. One white man with a burly chest and old aviator glasses jerked his torso toward us, his lower jaw jutting to the side. As we handed him a pipe, he explained, "I just got out of jail three days ago. For shooting a man. The bullet passed three inches from his heart. I'm lucky he didn't die, or I would have been in there a lot longer. Still, that was a year of my life. I'm going to get my life back together." I imagined that would be a lot easier to do if he had a place to call home.

One woman informed us about the "uranium messages" coming to her through the TV before adding a prescient point—"Better hopped up on meth than asleep and assaulted"—ending with a dry laugh. Over the years that followed, I would hear this explanation repeatedly from my patients. Many unhoused people who used meth did so only because they wanted to stay up longer to guard their possessions against theft and their body against assault; it wasn't a drug they actually liked to use.

Almost everyone thanked us with a closing line I didn't hear too often: "God bless." Some of our most popular items were purple nitrile gloves; people explained that they used them to pick up and throw away used needles. "There are kids out here, you know."

As night blanketed us in darkness, one man mistook us for a dealer, excitedly asking if we had any ice. "No, sorry, man," Joby responded. Nor did we have any more pipes, as almost every single person had wanted one. I was shocked. Perhaps I had expected half of the park's community to be using, but everyone? But, as studies suggested that substance use disorder was ten times more prevalent among adults experiencing homelessness compared to the general population, perhaps I shouldn't have been surprised.[4] Although the research isn't definitive as to whether substance use leads to homelessness or vice versa, as it is more likely a complicated and interrelated series of events responsible for both, it is clear that sustained recovery is nearly impossible without housing.[5]

As we finished up our loop and headed back to his car, it was ten till eight. "What did you think?" Joby asked.

"I was shocked how many people needed supplies." We followed a sidewalk under the glow of a streetlight.

"Yeah," he answered. "It's really hard to get syringes. The two county exchange programs recently shut down with no advance notice. One because of COVID, the other because somebody overdosed on-site, even though it was reversed with naloxone. Anyway." He flipped up his hands. "People basically don't have any way to get clean syringes right now. Last week when I came, people kept telling me, 'Oh, man, it's too bad you didn't come yesterday. We didn't have any syringes, so we were all sharing.'" He combed his fingers through his hair, shaking his head. "The only formal program left is at the Southern Arizona AIDS Foundation, but they require an exchange. In order to get a fresh syringe, you have to bring them a used one. But people don't want to carry used syringes around. It's illegal. I had a homie get arrested and go to jail for a year because of a dirty syringe. They weigh how much drug residue is left inside. A homie." He looked down at the ground as he walked, his long hair framing his pale face.

"What about pharmacies? Can people buy syringes there?"

"Yeah, theoretically, but most of the pharmacies won't sell to people who look like they might use drugs." Although it was legal for pharmacists to sell syringes without a prescription in Arizona, it was also a felony to distribute syringes to someone for the purpose of using drugs. Once again, the pharmacists had been scared away from treating addiction.

Out here in the park, it all seemed crazy, so cruel. Of course, I had read newspaper and journal articles about all these policies, but seeing how they played out in the lives of actual people was something else entirely. It felt less abstract, less theoretical. And none of it accidental.

Gazing at the stars overhead, I imagined another possible future. One in which people weren't arrested for possession of syringes or drugs, starting the cycle of homelessness and incarceration. Those simple interventions would probably reduce much of the chaotic drug use that seemed so prevalent. And for the rest, we could offer harm reduction—clean syringes and pipes instead of sharing, naloxone to reverse overdoses, and low barrier access to methadone and buprenorphine. I imagined a world in which methadone could be prescribed by any provider and picked up at any pharmacy, just as Marie wanted.

Over the past few years, users and activists have been some of methadone reform's staunchest advocates. During the beginning of the pandemic, the Urban Survivors Union wrote a statement demanding increased access to methadone via increased take-homes and reduced in-person requirements.[6] The statement was signed by over one hundred organizations, including the Harm Reduction Coalition, and received media coverage in *Time* and *Rolling Stone*. Marie would have been proud.

Following their lead, the American Society of Addiction Medicine, the American College of Academic Addiction Medicine, and other medical societies signed an open letter supporting the Modernizing Opioid Treatment Access Act (MOTAA), a bill that would expand methadone access.[7] However, I would argue that the proposed changes are still too small, as it limits methadone prescribing to board-certified addiction physicians, and there just aren't enough of us out there.[8] Additionally, the professional society that primarily represents methadone clinics, the American Association for the Treatment of Opioid Dependence, is staunchly against MOTAA.[9] Is it any coincidence that they might lose a revenue stream if their patients can obtain methadone from other doctors and pharmacies? Interestingly, their critiques of MOTAA repeat the same claims from the congressional hearings of the 1970s about the dangers of diversion. Will history repeat itself again?

Recently, harm reduction activists developed another innovative intervention to quell our country's overdose epidemic: supervised consumption sites, also known as overdose-prevention centers, where people can use drugs in a monitored setting. In many ways, they are a lot like bars. But, unlike bars, supervised consumption sites have staff trained in overdose reversal and linkage to care, distribute harm reduction supplies, and are often situated alongside MOUD clinics for those who become interested in treatment. In 2020, *The New England Journal of Medicine* published a study about an "unsanctioned safe consumption site" in an "undisclosed city" that local activists opened in 2014.[10] Over five years, people injected 10,514 times, and, although there were 33 opioid over-doses, all were successfully reversed by staff. Nobody needed to be transferred to an emergency department, and nobody died. It was a success. Studies of safe consumption sites internationally have also shown positive results.[11] This is the future we need, and it is being shaped and propelled forward by users themselves, not physicians. Unfortunately, when organizations tried to open sanctioned sites in San Francisco and Philadelphia, they were quickly shut down under 21 USC § 856—that is, the crack house statute. We still have so far to go.

But, thanks to researching this book, I at least have a framework for analyzing every "new" solution that a politician proposes to end overdose deaths: Does it treat addiction like a crime or a medical condition? Is it focused on the supply or the demand? Is it rooted in stigma or the humanity of people who use drugs? And did people who use drugs have a seat at the table?

When I said goodbye to Joby beside the mountains backlit by a rising moon, I did not yet know what the months and years ahead would hold: that I would give birth to a sweet spirit, finally find the supportive team I had been searching for among the addiction med-icine community in Tucson, become the director of our hospital's addiction medicine consult service, join the board of Cochise Harm Reduction, and lecture to hundreds of doctors about harm reduc-tion and addiction at national conferences, just like Marie. I would watch as the culture around addiction changed at my hospital, with more doctors and nurses eager to start MOUD and practice harm reduction. Together, we would apply for grants, reduce barriers to care, implement innovative programs, and publish our research. The needle was definitely moving, just slower than I would have liked.

I would also learn to practice radical empathy with my colleagues. When the Michigan ASAM president and I began to work together on various national committees, she apologized for not talking with me when the medical board investigation occurred. In her role as a board member, she had been instructed not to respond to any phy-sicians who contacted her about active investigations—she wasn't trying to be a jerk. Behind the scenes, she was actively working to make buprenorphine more accessible, including eliminating Michigan's additional licensure requirements. When I realized that not everyone was trying to betray me or people who used drugs, I didn't feel so alone.

With the help of harm reduction, I would grow more comfortable walking the narrow line between working from within the system and from outside it. I did not want to squander my opportunity to advocate from within the house of medicine, as my professional credentials gave me access and credibility in a way that many people who used drugs did not have. But, to appropriately steer my actions, I had to keep one foot planted in the grassroots of harm reduction, listening to users' priorities and paying attention to their solutions. In addition to this approach being more effective, it also resisted the prevailing doctor-as-savior trope I found so problematic. Even the democratic and decentralized structure of grassroots organizing was aspirational, offering an alternative to the racist hierarchy that had shaped our country's drug policy over the last century.

Similarly, my path to success did not need to perfectly follow Marie's. I didn't need to develop some groundbreaking new treatment. I didn't need to be seen as the expert. Such a shift in expectations carried with it a sense of ease; I no longer had to hold myself responsible for keeping a sinking boat afloat. I could only do what I could do. And we would do it together.

All of that is to say that the following years solidified a belief that sprouted that night out in the park with Joby: that if we want to heal our communities and end our country's overdose epidemic once and for all, harm reduction must be the foundation upon which everything else is built. Harm reduction, both as philosophy and as praxis, was the missing piece that Dorothy, Marie, and I had all been searching for, and it was Marie who led me here. In searching to understand a life from the past, I stumbled upon a better path for the future.

ACKNOWLEDGMENTS

Warren Greco, thank you for the boundless encouragement, the time you provided for me to write, and for being my first reader. Girls, part of the reason I wanted to write a book about a strong woman was for you. I hope that this book provides inspiration and fortitude, and that my career can make this world a little easier and brighter for you as you grow into women yourselves. Saudade Terán López, thank you for providing the space and support I needed for this book to take form. The same goes to our girls' caregivers and teachers at Kol Ami, Second Street School, Jardín de Niños Mi Tobogán, and Sam Hughes Elementary—quality childcare is rarely given the appreciation it deserves, but, without it, I couldn't have done any of this. I also want to thank my friends who let me vent while also encouraging me to listen to my heart.

If it weren't for Dr. Pamela Schaff, the physician whose narrative medicine course at the University of Southern California School of Medicine got me writing again; Dr. Paul Blackburn, one of my mentors at the Maricopa Emergency Medicine residency and a fervent practitioner of narrative medicine; and Dr. Karl Sporer, my fellowship mentor who encouraged me to pursue a master of fine arts in creative writing, I would not be here today.

For everyone who graciously gave me the time of day, suffered through my interviews, and trusted me with Marie, thank you: Dr. David Courtwright, Dr. Jerome Jaffe, Dr. Robert DuPont, Dr. Joyce Lowinson, and Paul Brodeur (may he rest in peace). Dr. Emily

Dufton, thanks for being my partner in the elite Marie Nyswander fan club.

My career in addiction medicine was largely shaped by the giants before me: Josh Luftig, Dr. Andrew Herring, Dr. Larry Oñate, Dr. Elissa Gumm, Dr. Cara Poland, Dr. Elizabeth Samuels, Dr. Gail D'Onofrio—thank you for your guidance. To all the visionary and dedicated harm reduction badasses—Lu Funk, Angel Gold, Samantha Childs, Haley Coles, Christopher Thomas, Joby—thank you for making such a difference in this world, educating me, and letting me hang out with you! And, of course, I want to thank my patients.

I also want to thank my EMS colleagues in Santa Cruz County who pushed for our leave-behind naloxone program (the first in the state!) and have kept the momentum going—Chief Jeffery Sargent, Chief Christian Renteria, Chief Jeff Polcari, Gerry Castro, and Chief Ben Guerrero—as well as my colleagues at the Arizona Department of Health Services and the University of Arizona Division of EMS who supported our efforts, including Dr. Gail Bradley, Ariel Moreno, Jacqueline Kurth, Sebastian Thomas, Milton Lerman, and Dr. Joshua Gaither. I also appreciate the support from Dr. José Cabañas, the president of the National Association of EMS Physicians who has uplifted the role of EMS in responding to our country's opioid epidemic, and the physician researchers who have collaborated with me on several projects, including Dr. Elizabeth Samuels, Dr. Anjni Joiner, Dr. Mary Mercer, Dr. Gene Hern, Dr. Remle Crowe, and Dr. Gerard Carroll.

At Mills College, I very much appreciated the forward-thinking pedagogy and the careful attention paid to my writing by professors Dr. Elmaz Abinader, Patricia Powell, Aamina Ahmad, and Kathryn Reiss during my MFA. They helped me transform a tangle of loose ideas into a thesis, which then transformed into this book.

Without my writing community—Heather Aruffo, Carli Cutchin, and Katie Lee Ellison from Jeannie Vanasco's nonfiction course at the Tin House Summer Workshop; Margo Steines, Natalie Lima, and Maya Bernstein-Schalet from the University of Arizona MFA program; Harmony Hazard and the Tucson-based Never Write Alone group; Erin Kannan; and my Pen Parentis writing accountability group (Laura Wheatman Hill, Jessica Manack, Isabel Choi,

Carolyn Silveira, Lisa Gouldy, Billy Kilgore, Jana-Lee Blaish, Melissa Bandy, Kate Blakinger, and Lane Igoudin)—I probably would have fallen into a state of despondent loneliness. I also want to thank those writers whose hybrid memoirs inspired my own, especially Daisy Hernández and Jenn Shapland. Ander Monson and Francisco Cantú, thanks for letting me take nonfiction workshops at the University of Arizona. Jill Christman and Todd McKinney—thank you for believing in my related essay at *River Teeth*. I very much appreciated the inspiration and space to write granted by the Casa Lü Sur residency in Mexico City (Guadalupe Quesada, Vicente Quesada, Michele Saenz, Mireya Lastiri, Mariana Lagort, Amado Cabrales, Nabil Yanai Salazar Sánchez, Carolina Velez Muñiz, and Hannah Villanueva) and the financial support from the Arizona Commission on the Arts.

Thank you, Liz Gassman, for your astute proposal edits. I also very much appreciate my agent, Ayla Zuraw-Friedland, who took me in from the slush pile and carefully crafted the shape of my book into something much better, and my editor at Beacon, Haley Lynch, who gave me the advice I needed while also respecting my vision, elevating this project to the next level. To the entire Beacon team, including Gayatri Patnaik, Susan Lumenello, Marcy Barnes, Alyssa Hassan, Bev Rivero, Frankie Karnedy, and everyone else behind the scenes—thank you for supporting my debut and crafting it into a beautiful, final product. Thank you, Cassie Mannes Murray, for helping to get my work further into the world.

NOTES

CHAPTER 1: THE CLINIC

1. Department of Health and Human Services, "Medications for the Treatment of Opioid Use Disorder," https://public-inspection.federalregister.gov/2024-01693.pdf, accessed September 30, 2024.

2. Judith E. Tintinalli et al., *Tintinalli's Emergency Medicine: A Comprehensive Study Guide*, 8th ed. (McGraw-Hill Education, 2016).

3. CASA Columbia National Advisory Commission on Addiction Treatment, *Addiction Medicine: Closing the Gap Between Science and Practice*, June 2012, https://www.hr-dp.org/files/2015/07/13/Addiction-medicine-closing-the-gap-between-science-and-practice_(1).pdf.

4. CASA Columbia National Advisory Commission on Addiction Treatment, *Addiction Medicine*.

5. Office of the Surgeon General, *Facing Addiction in America: The Surgeon General's Spotlight on Opioids* (US Department of Health and Human Services, September 2018).

6. CASA Columbia National Advisory Commission on Addiction Treatment, *Addiction Medicine*.

7. R. Ries, D. Fiellin, S. Miller, R. Sait, eds., *The ASAM Principles of Addiction Medicine*, 5th ed. (Wolters Kluwer, 2014), 4.

8. American Psychiatric Association, *Diagnostic and Statistical Manual of Mental Disorders*, 5th ed. (American Psychiatric Publishing, 2013).

9. N. Volkow and K. Warren, "Drug Addiction: The Neurobiology of Behavior Gone Awry," in Ries et al., *The ASAM Principles of Addiction Medicine*, 4–9.

10. S. R. Dube et al., "Childhood Abuse, Neglect, and Household Dysfunction and the Risk of Illicit Drug Use: The Adverse Childhood Experiences Study," *Pediatrics* 111, no. 3 (March 2003): 564–72, doi: 10.1542/peds.111.3.564.

11. B. M. Kuehn, "Methadone Treatment Marks 40 Years," *Journal of the American Medical Association (JAMA)* 294, no. 8 (August 2005): 887–89, doi: 10.1001/jama.294.8.887.

12. V. P. Dole and M. Nyswander, "A Medical Treatment for Diacetylmorphine (Heroin) Addiction: A Clinical Trial with Methadone Hydrochloride," *JAMA* 193 (August 1965): 646–50, doi: 10.1001/jama.1965.03090080008002.

13. Kuehn, "Methadone Treatment Marks 40 Years."

14. Centers for Disease Control and Prevention, *Module 5: Assessing and Addressing Opioid Use Disorder*, WB 2863, updated June 12, 2018, https://www.cdc.gov/drugoverdose/training/oud/accessible/index.html.

15. NIDA, "Drug Overdose Death Rates," June 30, 2023, https://nida.nih.gov/research-topics/trends-statistics/overdose-death-rates.

16. David Courtwright, notes on transcription of interview with Charlie Winick, January 25, 1993.

CHAPTER 2: THE BEGINNING

1. Nat Hentoff, *A Doctor Among the Addicts* (Rand McNally, 1968), 59.

2. Marie Nyswander, interview with David Courtwright, June 22, 1981.

3. M. Nyswander, interview.

4. Hentoff, *A Doctor Among the Addicts*.

5. Joshua Clark Davis, "The Forgotten World of Communist Bookstores," *Jacobin*, August 11, 2017, https://jacobinmag.com/2017/08/communist-party-cpusa-bookstore-fbi.

6. *New York Times*, Reds Try to Stir Negroes to Revolt, July 28, 1919; Robert K. Murray, *Red Scare: A Study in National Hysteria, 1919–1920* (University of Minnesota, 1955), p. 57–58, 119–121, 214–222; Robert Justin Goldstein, ed., *Little "Red Scares": Anti-Communism and Political Repression in the United States, 1921–1946* (Ashgate, 2014).

7. Dale Mineshima-Lowe, "Criminal Syndicalism Laws," *The First Amendment Encyclopedia*, Free Speech Center, Middle Tennessee State University, January 1, 2009, https://www.mtsu.edu/first-amendment/article/942/criminal-syndicalism-laws.

8. Hentoff, *A Doctor Among the Addicts*.

9. M. Nyswander, interview.

10. Nancy Campbell, *OD: Naloxone and the Politics of Overdose* (MIT Press, 2020).

11. M. Nyswander, interview.

12. Editorial Staff, "Job Hunting Hard on Faith but Eventful to Faith Too," *The Campus*, October 23, 1940.

13. Mr. Hormel of the Hormel Ham Corporation.

14. United Press, "Jap Silk Feeds Student Bonfire," *Cleveland Plain Dealer*, December 31, 1938.

15. Jennifer Harlan and Veronica Chambers, "First Inklings of Fame," *New York Times*, September 18, 2020, https://www.nytimes.com/2020/05/22/us/first-photos-celebrities-graduation.html.

16. Harlan and Chambers, "First Inklings of Fame."

17. "She Wants to Be a Lion or What Are Suppressed Desires?" *The Campus*, December 13, 1939.

18. Dorothy Nyswander, interview with David Courtwright, February 17, 1992.

19. M. Nyswander, interview.

20. "History of Women in Medicine," Office for Diversity and Inclusion, Heersink School of Medicine, University of Alabama at Birmingham, https://

www.uab.edu/medicine/diversity/initiatives/women/history, accessed August 2021, available at https://web.archive.org/web/20230325133823/https:/www .uab.edu/medicine/diversity/initiatives/women/history.

21. Hentoff, *A Doctor Among the Addicts*.

22. M. Nyswander, interview.

23. "Intra-Views," *Sarah Lawrence College Alumnae Magazine*, 1947, 19–20.

24. Personal communication with David Courtwright, 2021.

25. A. Dayal et al., "Comparison of Male vs. Female Resident Milestone Evaluations by Faculty During Emergency Medicine Residency Training," *JAMA Internal Medicine* 177, no. 5 (May 2017): 651–57.

26. A. Espaillat et al., "An Exploratory Study on Microaggressions in Medical School: What Are They and Why Should We Care?" *Perspectives on Medical Education* 8, no. 3 (June 2019): 143–51, doi: 10.1007/s40037-019-0516-3.

27. M. I. O'Connor, "Medical School Experiences Shape Women Students' Interest in Orthopaedic Surgery," *Clinical Orthopaedics and Related Research* 474, no. 9 (September 2016): 1967–72, doi: 10.1007/s11999-016-4830-3.

28. Dayal et al., "Comparison of Male vs. Female Resident Milestone Evaluations by Faculty During Emergency Medicine Residency Training."

29. A. S. Mueller et al., "Gender Differences in Attending Physicians' Feedback to Residents: A Qualitative Analysis," *Journal of Graduate Medical Education* 9, no. 5 (2017): 577–85, doi: 10.4300/JGME-D-17-00126.1.

30. S. L. Galvin et al., "Gender Bias in Nurse Evaluations of Residents in Obstetrics and Gynecology," *Obstetrics & Gynecology* 126, Suppl. 4 (2015): 7S–12S, doi: 10.1097/AOG.0000000000001044.

31. S. Koven, "Letter to a Young Female Physician," *New England Journal of Medicine* 376, no. 20 (May 18, 2017): 1907–9, doi: 10.1056/NEJMp1702010.

32. Y. Tsugawa et al., "Comparison of Hospital Mortality and Readmission Rates for Medicare Patients Treated by Male vs. Female Physicians," *JAMA Internal Medicine* 177, no. 2 (2017): 206–13, doi:10.1001/jamainternmed .2016.7875

33. "Intra-Views," *Sarah Lawrence College Alumnae Magazine*, 1947, 19–20.

CHAPTER 3: BUPISTA

1. By Dr. Kathy LeSaint.

2. Abby Goodnough, "E.R. Treats Opioid Addiction on Demand. That's Very Rare," *New York Times*, August 18, 2018, https://www.nytimes.com/2018/08 /18/health/opioid-addiction-treatment.html.

3. On January 12, 2023, SAMHSA and the DEA issued guidance on the removal of the x-waiver: https://www.deadiversion.usdoj.gov/pubs/docs/A-23 -0020-Dear-Registrant-Letter-Signed.pdf.

4. J. Netherland and H. White, "Opioids: Pharmaceutical Race and the War on Drugs That Wasn't," *Biosocieties* 12, no. 2 (June 2017): 217–38, doi: 10.1057 /biosoc.2015.46.

5. N. J. Kazerouni et al., "Pharmacy-Related Buprenorphine Access Barriers: An Audit of Pharmacies in Counties with a High Opioid Overdose Burden,"

Drug and Alcohol Dependence 224, no. 108729 (July 1, 2021), doi: 10.1016/j .drugalcdep.2021.108729.

6. H. L. F. Cooper et al., "When Prescribing Isn't Enough—Pharmacy-Level Barriers to Buprenorphine Access," *New England Journal of Medicine* 383, no. 8 (August 20, 2020): 703–5, doi: 10.1056/NEJMp2002908.

7. J. Bruneau et al., "Management of Opioid Use Disorders: A National Clinical Practice Guideline," *CMAJ* 190, no. 9 (March 5, 2018): E247–57, doi: 10.1503/cmaj.170958.

8. Marie Nyswander, *The Drug Addict as a Patient* (Grune & Stratton, 1956).

9. Center for Drug Evaluation and Research (CDER) World Training, *Pediatric Drug Development*, FDA, https://www.accessdata.fda.gov/scripts/cderworld /index.cfm, accessed May 1, 2021.

10. David Musto, *The American Disease: Origins of Narcotic Control* (Oxford University Press, 1973).

11. *Examiner* Staff, "The Country's First War on Drugs: SF vs. Opium," *San Francisco Examiner*, June 11, 2015, https://www.sfexaminer.com/news/the -countrys-first-war-on-drugs-sf-vs-opium/.

12. Edward Breecher and *Consumer Reports Magazine*, "Opium Smoking Is Outlawed," in *The Consumers Union Report on Licit and Illicit Drugs*, 1972, https://www.druglibrary.org/schaffer/library/studies/cu/cu6.htm, accessed May 1, 2021; Charles Terry and Mildred Pellens, *The Opium Problem* (Patterson Smith, 1928), 73.

13. Musto, *The American Disease*, 6.

14. *Examiner* Staff, "The Country's First War on Drugs."

15. Benson Tong, *The Chinese Americans* (Greenwood Press, 2000), 81.

16. Jefferson M. Fish, *How to Legalize Drugs* (Jason Aronson, 1998), 244; Johann Hari, *Chasing the Scream: The Search for the Truth About Addiction* (Bloomsbury, 2015), 28.

17. Musto, *The American Disease*, 7.

18. Musto, *The American Disease*, 6.

19. Musto, *The American Disease*, 7.

20. Musto, *The American Disease*.

21. Breecher and *Consumer Reports Magazine*, "Opium Smoking Is Outlawed."

22. Harrison Narcotics Act, Public Law No. 223, 63rd Cong., approved December 17, 1914.

23. New York Medical Journal, "Mental Sequelae of the Harrison Law," 102 (May 15, 1915): 1014; Breecher and *Consumer Reports Magazine*, "Opium Smoking Is Outlawed."

24. Musto, *The American Disease*, 107.

25. Musto, *The American Disease*, 123.

26. Breecher and *Consumer Reports Magazine*, "Opium Smoking Is Outlawed."

27. Musto, *The American Disease*, 92, 107.

28. Musto, *The American Disease*, 108.

29. Hearings Before the Subcommittee to Investigate Juvenile Delinquency of the Committee on the Judiciary, United States Senate, Ninety-Fourth Congress Second Session, *Investigation of Juvenile Delinquency in the United*

States. Narcotic Sentencing and Seizure Act of 1976, vol. 1, July 28 and August 5, 1976, p. 721.

30. US Circuit Court of Appeals, Sixth Circuit, No. 3068, W. S. Webb and Jacob Goldbaum, *Plaintiffs in Error v. United States of America,* Defendant in Error, Filed February 11, 1918, by Win C. Cochran, Clerk.

31. Musto, *The American Disease,* 140.

32. L. Malichi Harney, "Trial and Failure of the Ambulatory Treatment of (Opiate) Drug Addiction in the United States," January 1, 1964, https://www .unodc.org/unodc/en/data-and-analysis/bulletin/bulletin_1964-01-01_2 _page004.html.

33. Nyswander, *The Drug Addict as a Patient.*

34. Nyswander, *The Drug Addict as a Patient.*

35. Nyswander, *The Drug Addict as a Patient.*

36. Marie Nyswander, interview with David Courtwright, June 22, 1981.

CHAPTER 4: NARCO

1. Nat Hentoff, *A Doctor Among the Addicts* (Rand McNally, 1968), 63.

2. Marie Nyswander, interview by David Courtwright, June 22, 1981.

3. B. Murphy, "These Medical Specialties Have the Biggest Gender Imbalances," American Medical Association, October 1, 2019, https://www.ama-assn .org/residents-students/specialty-profiles/these-medical-specialties-have -biggest-gender-imbalances.

4. "Intra-Views," *Sarah Lawrence College Alumnae Magazine,* 1947, 19–20.

5. Leslie Jamison, *The Recovering: Intoxication and Its Aftermath* (Little, Brown, 2018).

6. Nancy D. Campbell, J. P. Olsen, and Luke Walden, *The Narcotic Farm: The Rise and Fall of America's First Prison for Drug Addicts* (University Press of Kentucky/South Limestone, 2021).

7. Nancy Campbell, *OD: Naloxone and the Politics of Overdose* (MIT Press, 2020).

8. William S. Burroughs, *Junky* (Penguin, 1977).

9. C. G. Leukefeld and F. M. Tims, eds., *Compulsory Treatment of Drug Abuse: Research and Clinical Practice,* National Institute on Drug Abuse, 1988; Marjorie Senechal, "Narco Brat," in *Of Human Bondage: Historical Perspectives on Addiction,* ed. Douglas L. Patey, *Smith College Studies in History* 52 (Smith College, 2003), 173–200, https://www.addiction-ssa.org/wp-content/uploads /2019/11/NarcoBrat.pdf.

10. Maia Szalavitz, "Why Forced Addiction Treatment Fails," *New York Times,* April 30, 2022, https://www.nytimes.com/2022/04/30/opinion/forced -addiction-treatment.html.

11. D. Werb et al., "The Effectiveness of Compulsory Drug Treatment: A Systematic Review," *International Journal of Drug Policy* 28 (February 2016): 1–9, doi: 10.1016/j.drugpo.2015.12.005.

12. C. Rafful et al., "Increased Non-Fatal Overdose Risk Associated with Involuntary Drug Treatment in a Longitudinal Study with People Who Inject Drugs," *Addiction* 113, no. 6 (June 2018): 1056–63, doi: 10.1111/add.14159.

13. Leukefeld and Tims, *Compulsory Treatment of Drug Abuse*.

14. Jamison, *The Recovering*.

15. Senechal, "Narco Brat."

16. Campbell, Olsen, and Walden, *The Narcotic Farm*.

17. Michelle Alexander, *The New Jim Crow: Mass Incarceration in the Age of Colorblindness* (New Press, 2010.)

18. Alexander, *The New Jim Crow*; Marc Mauer and Sentencing Project, *Race to Incarcerate*, rev. ed. (New Press, 2006), 33; Human Rights Watch, *Punishment and Prejudice: Racial Disparities in the War on Drugs*, HRW Reports 12, no. 2 (New York, 2000); US Bureau of Justice Statistics, "Prisoners in 2022—Statistical Tables," November 2023, https://bjs.ojp.gov/document/p22st.pdf, p. 34.

19. World Prison Brief, "Highest to Lowest—Prison Population Rate," https://www.prisonstudies.org/highest-to-lowest/prison_population_rate, accessed August 30, 2024.

20. SAMHSA, "Highlights by Race/Ethnicity for the 2023 National Survey on Drug Use and Health," https://www.samhsa.gov/data/sites/default/files/NSDUH%202023%20Annual%20Release/2023-nsduh-race-eth-highlights.pdf, accessed November 1, 2024; L. J. Floyd et al., "Adolescent Drug Dealing and Race/Ethnicity: A Population-Based Study of the Differential Impact of Substance Use on Involvement in Drug Trade," *American Journal of Drug and Alcohol Abuse* 36, no. 2 (March 2010): 87–91, doi: 10.3109/00952991003587469; Human Rights Watch, *Punishment and Prejudice*.

21. Human Rights Watch, *Punishment and Prejudice*.

22. Merianne Rose Spencer et al., "Data Brief 457; Drug Overdose Deaths in the United States, 2001–2021," Centers for Disease Control and Prevention, https://www.cdc.gov/nchs/data/databriefs/db457-tables.pdf#4, accessed November 1, 2024.

23. National Center for Health Statistics, "U.S. Overdose Deaths Decrease in 2023, First Time Since 2018," press release, CDC, May 15, 2024, https://www.cdc.gov/nchs/pressroom/nchs_press_releases/2024/20240515.htm.

24. Campbell, Olsen, and Walden, *The Narcotic Farm*.

25. Senechal, "Narco Brat."

26. Campbell, Olsen, and Walden, *The Narcotic Farm*.

27. David Courtwright, *Dark Paradise: A History of Opiate Addiction in America* (Harvard University Press, 2001).

28. Johann Hari, *Chasing the Scream: The Search for the Truth About Addiction* (Bloomsbury, 2015).

29. David T. Courtwright, Herman Joseph, and Don Des Jarlais, *Addicts Who Survived: An Oral History of Narcotic Use in America, 1923–1965* (University of Tennessee Press, 1989).

30. Hari, *Chasing the Scream*, 19.

31. The research unit may not have been in a separate building during Marie's time; she described it as being in the bowels of the building in Hentoff's biography (66).

32. It was not called this officially until 1948.

33. Marie Nyswander, *The Drug Addict as a Patient* (Grune & Stratton, 1956).

34. R. J. Defalque and A. J. Wright, "The Early History of Methadone: Myths and Facts," *Bulletin of Anesthesia History* 25, no. 3 (October 2007): 13–16, doi: 10.1016/s1522-8649(07)50035-1.

35. F. López-Muñoz et al., "The Pharmaceutical Industry and the German National Socialist Regime: I. G. Farben and Pharmacological Research," *Journal of Clinical Pharmacy and Therapeutics* 34, no. 1 (February 2009): 67–77, doi: 10.1111/j.1365-2710.2008.00972.x.

36. Defalque and Wright, "The Early History of Methadone."

37. H. Isbell et al., "Tolerance and Addiction Liability of 6-Dimethylamino-4-4-Diphenylheptanone-3 (Methadon)," *JAMA* 135, no. 14 (December 6, 1947): 888–94, doi: 10.1001/jama.1947.02890140008003.

38. Stacey Pauker, "From Protectionism to Access: Women's Participation in Clinical Trials—Conflict, Controversy, and Change," April 2002, https://dash .harvard.edu/bitstream/handle/1/8889449/Pauker.html.

39. Harriet Washington, *Medical Apartheid: The Dark History of Medical Experimentation on Black Americans from Colonial Times to the Present* (Anchor, 2006), 258–59.

40. Jean Heller, "AP Was There: Black Men Untreated in Tuskegee Syphilis Study," AP News, May 10, 2017, https://apnews.com/article/business-science -health-race-and-ethnicity-syphilis-e9dd07eaa4e74052878a68132cd3803a.

41. Campbell, Olsen, and Walden, *The Narcotic Farm.*

42. Campbell, Olsen, and Walden, *The Narcotic Farm.*

43. Nyswander, *The Drug Addict as a Patient.*

44. *The Distant Drummer: Bridge from No Place*, aka *Bridge from No Place*, dir. William Templeton, National Institute of Mental Health, 1971, http:// resource.nlm.nih.gov/101299851.

45. Campbell, Olsen, and Walden, *The Narcotic Farm.*

46. Campbell, Olsen, and Walden, *The Narcotic Farm.*

47. Campbell, *OD.*

48. Nyswander, *The Drug Addict as a Patient.*

49. Isbell et al., "Tolerance and Addiction Liability of 6-Dimethylamino-4-4-Diphenylheptanone-3 (Methadon)."

50. I believe, based on the dates and documentation, that she learned about methadone at Narco.

51. V. H. Vogel et al., "Present Status of Narcotic Addiction with Particular Reference to Medical Indications and Comparative Addiction Liability of the Newer and Older Analgesic Drugs," *JAMA* 138, no. 14 (December 4, 1948): 1019–26, doi: 10.1001/jama.1948.02900140011003.

52. Nyswander, *The Drug Addict as a Patient.*

53. Senechal, "Narco Brat."

54. Hentoff, *A Doctor Among the Addicts.*

55. M. Nyswander, interview.

56. Hentoff, *A Doctor Among the Addicts*, 64.

57. M. Nyswander, interview.

58. Hentoff, *A Doctor Among the Addicts*, 66.

59. Hentoff, *A Doctor Among the Addicts*, 71.

60. Senechal, "Narco Brat."

61. Hentoff, *A Doctor Among the Addicts,* 66.

62. M. Nyswander, interview.

63. Hentoff, *A Doctor Among the Addicts,* 64.

64. M. Nyswander, interview.

CHAPTER 5: FLIGHT

1. Renate Ysseldyk et al., "A Leak in the Academic Pipeline: Identity and Health Among Postdoctoral Women," *Frontiers in Psychology* 10 (March 3, 2019), https://www.frontiersin.org/journals/psychology/articles/10.3389/fpsyg .2019.01297/full.

2. Erin Zimmerman, *Unrooted: Botany, Motherhood, and the Fight to Save an Old Science* (Melville House, 2024).

3. A. Y. Walley et al., "Opioid Overdose Rates and Implementation of Overdose Education and Nasal Naloxone Distribution in Massachusetts: Interrupted Time Series Analysis," *British Medical Journal* 346, no. f174 (January 30, 2013), doi: 10.1136/bmj.f174.

4. K. H. Seal et al., "Naloxone Distribution and Cardiopulmonary Resuscitation Training for Injection Drug Users to Prevent Heroin Overdose Death: A Pilot Intervention Study," *Journal of Urban Health* 82, no. 2 (2005): 303–11; K. D. Wagner et al., "Evaluation of an Overdose Prevention and Response Training Programme for Injection Drug Users in the Skid Row Area of Los Angeles, CA," *International Journal of Drug Policy* 21, no. 3 (2010): 186–93; M. Doe-Simkins et al., "Overdose Rescues by Trained and Untrained Participants and Change in Opioid Use Among Substance Using Participants in Overdose Education and Naloxone Distribution Programs: A Retrospective Cohort Study," *BMC Public Health* 14 (2014): 297.

5. North American Syringe Exchange Network (NASEN).

6. Corey Davis, "Overdose 'Good Samaritan' Laws Should Protect, Not Punish," Network for Public Health Law, January 26, 2020, https://www.network forphl.org/news-insights/overdose-good-samaritan-laws-should-protect-not -punish/.

7. Maia Szalavitz, *Undoing Drugs: How Harm Reduction Is Changing the Future of Drugs and Addiction* (New York: Hachette, 2021).

8. H. E. Tookes et al., "A Comparison of Syringe Disposal Practices Among Injection Drug Users in a City with Versus a City Without Needle and Syringe Programs," *Drug and Alcohol Dependence* 123, no. 1–3 (2012): 255–59, doi: 10.1016/j.drugalcdep.2011.12.001.

9. World Health Organization, "Effectiveness of Sterile Needle and Syringe Programming in Reducing HIV/AIDS Among Injecting Drug Users," technical paper, 2004.

10. Center for Innovative Public Policies, "Needle Exchange Programs: Is Baltimore a Bust?" April 2001, 82–89.

11. S. L. Groseclose et al., "Impact of Increased Legal Access to Needles and Syringes on Practices of Injecting-Drug Users and Police Officers—Connecticut, 1992–1993," *Journal of Acquired Immune Deficiency Syndromes & Human Retrovirology* 1, no. 13 (September 1995): 82–89.

12. R. N. Bluthenthal et al., "Higher Syringe Coverage Is Associated with Lower Odds of HIV Risk and Does Not Increase Unsafe Syringe Disposal Among Syringe Exchange Program Clients," *Drug and Alcohol Dependence* 89, nos. 2–3 (2007): 214–22, doi: 10.1016/j.drugalcdep.2006.12.035.

13. Meg O'Connor, "'Nation's Only Female Chaingang' Apparently Disbanded," *Phoenix New Times*, May 2, 2019, https://www.phoenixnewtimes.com/news/nations-only-female-chain-gang-boasts-the-mcso-website-11279199.

14. SAMHSA, Center for Behavioral Health Statistics and Quality, National Survey on Drug Use and Health (NSDUH), 2015, https://www.samhsa.gov/data/sites/default/files/NSDUH-DetTabs-2015/NSDUH-DetTabs-2015/NSDUH-DetTabs-2015.pdf.

CHAPTER 6: ROPED BACK

1. "Bellevue Psychiatric Hospital," Asylum Projects, May 28, 2021, https://www.asylumprojects.org/index.php/Bellevue_Psychiatric_Hospital.

2. Marie Nyswander, interview by David Courtwright, June 22, 1981.

3. F. López-Muñoz et al., "The History of Barbiturates a Century After Their Clinical Introduction," *Neuropsychiatric Disease and Treatment* 1, no. 4 (2005): 329–43.

4. Marie Nyswander, "Withdrawal Treatment of Drug Addiction," *New England Journal of Medicine* 242, no. 4 (January 26, 1950): 128–30, doi: 10.1056/NEJM195001262420403.

5. M. Nyswander, interview.

6. Nyswander, "Withdrawal Treatment of Drug Addiction."

7. M. Nyswander, interview.

8. Nat Hentoff, *A Doctor Among the Addicts*, (Rand McNally, 1968), 69.

9. Hentoff, *A Doctor Among the Addicts*, 69.

10. M. Nyswander, interview.

11. This scene is imagined, but the scenario is described in Hentoff, *A Doctor Among the Addicts*, 69.

12. M. Nyswander et al., "Treatment of the Narcotic Addict: Workshop, 1957. 1. The Treatment of Drug Addicts as Voluntary Outpatients: A Progress Report," *American Journal of Orthopsychiatry* 4 (October 28, 1958): 714–27, discussion 727–29, doi: 10.1111/j.1939-0025.1958.tb03988.x.

13. Hentoff, *A Doctor Among the Addicts*, 70.

14. Hentoff, *A Doctor Among the Addicts*, 71.

15. M. Nyswander, interview.

16. Nancy Campbell, *OD: Naloxone and the Politics of Overdose* (MIT Press, 2020).

17. C. Budnick, H. Pickard, and W. White, *Narcotics Anonymous Chronology*, vol. 1, October 2013, https://www.chestnut.org/resources/7dc39aea-7864-43d0-904d-46db4fb9b946/2013-percent-20NA-percent-20Chronology-percent-20--percent-20Volume-percent-20One-percent-202nd-percent-20Edition.pdf.

18. M. Nyswander, interview.

19. Hentoff, *A Doctor Among the Addicts*, 71.

20. M. Nyswander et al., "Treatment of the Narcotic Addict."

21. M. Nyswander et al., "Treatment of the Narcotic Addict."

22. M. Nyswander, interview.

23. M. Nyswander, interview.

24. Johann Hari, *Chasing the Scream: The Search for the Truth About Addiction* (Bloomsbury, 2015).

25. Hari, *Chasing the Scream*, 18.

26. M. Nyswander, interview.

27. Hari, *Chasing the Scream*.

28. M. Nyswander, interview; scene imagined, text quoted.

29. Beatrice Berle, *A Life in Two Worlds: The Autobiography of Beatrice Bishop Berle* (Walker, 1983), 208.

30. Charles Winick, interview with David Courtwright, January 25, 1993.

31. B. B. Berle and M. Nyswander, "Ambulatory Withdrawal Treatment of Heroin Addicts," *New York State Journal of Medicine*, July 15, 1964.

32. M. Nyswander, interview.

33. Marie Nyswander, *The Drug Addict as a Patient* (Grune & Stratton, 1956).

34. David Musto, *The American Disease: Origins of Narcotic Control* (Oxford University Press, 1999).

35. Hentoff, *A Doctor Among the Addicts*, 28.

36. "Clinic vs. Prison," *Times-Picayune*, September 14, 1958.

37. Hentoff, *A Doctor Among the Addicts*, 111.

38. M. Nyswander, interview.

CHAPTER 7: SISYPHUS

1. G. D'Onofrio et al., "Emergency Department–Initiated Buprenorphine/Naloxone Treatment for Opioid Dependence: A Randomized Clinical Trial," *JAMA* 313, no. 16 (2015): 1636–44.

2. J. A. Hoppe et al., "Opioid Prescribing in a Cross Section of US Emergency Departments," *Annals of Emergency Medicine* 66 (2015): 253–59.

3. Hoppe et al., "Opioid Prescribing in a Cross Section of US Emergency Departments."

4. J. A. Hoppe et al., "Association of Emergency Department Opioid Initiation with Recurrent Opioid Use," *Annals of Emergency Medicine* 65 (2015): 493–99.

5. J. Bruneau et al., "Management of Opioid Use Disorders: A National Clinical Practice Guideline," *CMAJ* 190, no. 9 (March 5, 2018): E247–E257, doi: 10.1503/cmaj.170958.

6. J. Emmanuelli and J. C. Desenclos, "Harm Reduction Interventions, Behaviours and Associated Health Outcomes in France, 1996–2003," *Addiction* 100, no. 11 (November 2005): 1690–700, doi: 10.1111/j.1360-0443.2005.01271.x; erratum in *Addiction* 101, no. 4 (April 2006): 616, PMID: 16277629.

7. R. P. Schwartz et al., "Opioid Agonist Treatments and Heroin Overdose Deaths in Baltimore, Maryland, 1995–2009," *American Journal of Public Health* 103, no. 5 (May 2013): 917–22, doi: 10.2105/AJPH.2012.301049.

8. J. Kakko et al., "1-Year Retention and Social Function After Buprenorphine-Assisted Relapse Prevention Treatment for Heroin Dependence in Sweden: A Randomised, Placebo-Controlled Trial," *Lancet* 361, no. 9358 (February 22, 2003): 662–68, doi: 10.1016/S0140-6736(03)12600-1.

9. Rockefeller University, "Fifty Years After Landmark Methadone Discovery, Stigmas and Misunderstandings Persist," *Science News,* December 9, 2016, https://www.rockefeller.edu/news/12410-fifty-years-after-landmark-methadone-discovery-stigmas-and-misunderstandings-persist/.

10. K. Dugosh et al., "A Systematic Review on the Use of Psychosocial Interventions in Conjunction with Medications for the Treatment of Opioid Addiction," *Journal of Addiction Medicine* 10, no. 2 (2016): 93–103, doi: 10.1097/ADM.0000000000000193.

11. Ruben Strayer et al., "Management of Opioid Use Disorder in the Emergency Department: A White Paper Prepared for the American Academy of Emergency Medicine," https://www.aaem.org/UserFiles/file/AAEMOUDWhitePaperManuscript.pdf, accessed May 1, 2021.

12. L. Ti, "Leaving the Hospital Against Medical Advice Among People Who Use Illicit Drugs: A Systematic Review," *American Journal of Public Health* 105, no. 12 (2015): 53–59.

13. A. C. Chan et al., "HIV-Positive Injection Drug Users Who Leave the Hospital Against Medical Advice: The Mitigating Role of Methadone and Social Support," *Journal of Acquired Immune Deficiency Syndromes* 35, no. 1 (2004): 56–59.

14. Now we better understand the use of cross-tapers, so patients don't have to go through withdrawal first, but this practice still is the exception rather than the norm.

15. 21 C.F.R. § 1306.07 (b) and (c).

16. Robert Newman, interview with David Courtwright, July 24, 1981.

CHAPTER 8: THE CURE

1. Joyce Lowinson, interview with Melody Glenn, May 15, 2021.

2. Vincent Dole, interview with David Courtwright, September 13, 1982.

3. This was based on the British system.

4. Nat Hentoff, *A Doctor Among the Addicts* (Grove Press, 1968), 93.

5. Dole, interview.

6. Robert Newman, interview with David Courtwright, July 24, 1981.

7. Newman, interview.

8. Dole, interview.

9. NCHS, "Deaths and Mortality," CDC, https://www.cdc.gov/NCHS/fastats/deaths.htm, accessed November 1, 2024.

CHAPTER 10: ZENITH

1. Ray Trussell, interview with Herman Joseph, September 26, 1983.

2. Joyce Lowinson, interview with Melody Glenn, May 15, 2021.

3. William Farrell, "City Backs Plan to Cure Addicts," *New York Times,* June 8, 1965.

4. Morris Kaplan, "City Will Expand Methadone Test," *New York Times,* August 25, 1965.

5. Dr. Efrén/Ephraim Ramirez. He had even opened his own TC's in Puerto Rico. Beny J. Primm, *The Healer: A Doctor's Crusade Against Addiction and AIDS* (Create Space Independent Publishing Platform, 2014), 16.

6. NA World Services, *Narcotics Anonymous and Persons Receiving Medication-Assisted Treatment*, 2016, https://www.na.org/admin/include/spaw2 /uploads/pdf/pr/2306_NA_PRMAT_1021.pdf, accessed July 22, 2021.

7. Gertrude Samuels, "Methadone—Fighting Fire with Fire," *New York Times*, October 15, 1967.

8. Frances Gearing, interview with Herman Joseph, November 28, 1983.

9. Gearing, interview.

10. Gearing, interview.

11. Maia Szalavitz, *Undoing Drugs: How Harm Reduction Is Changing the Future of Drugs and Addiction* (Hachette, 2021), 52.

12. Methadone Maintenance Evaluation Committee, "Progress Report of Evaluation of Methadone Maintenance Treatment Program as of March 31, 1968," *JAMA* 206, no. 12 (December 16, 1968).

13. E. Ranzal, "City Plans to Double Methadone Project," *New York Times*, September 30, 1970.

14. In the 1968 Gallup poll, 81 percent of respondents agreed with the statement "Law and order has broken down in this country," and the majority blamed "Negroes who start riots" and "communists."

15. Michelle Alexander, *The New Jim Crow: Mass Incarceration in the Age of Colorblindness* (New Press, 2010), 45.

16. Dan Baum, *Smoke and Mirrors: The War on Drugs and the Politics of Failure* (Little, Brown, 1996).

17. Jerome Jaffe, interview, "Drug Wars," *Frontline*, PBS, 2000, https://www .pbs.org/wgbh/pages/frontline/shows/drugs/interviews/jaffe.html, accessed May 1, 2021.

18. Ranzal, "City Plans to Double Methadone Project."

19. Gearing, interview.

20. Jeffrey Donfeld, interview with Melody Glenn, June 17, 2021.

21. V. Dole et al., "Successful Treatment of 750 Criminal Addicts," *JAMA* 206 (1968): 2708–11.

22. C. K. Scott et al., "The Impact of the Opioid Crisis on U.S. State Prison Systems," *Health Justice* 24, no. 9 (July 24, 2021): 17, doi: 10.1186/s40352-021 -00143-9.

23. ACLU, *Over-Jailed and Un-Treated*, 2021, https://www.aclu.org/wp -content/uploads/publications/20210625-mat-prison_1.pdf, accessed November 1, 2024; National Institute on Drug Abuse, "Criminal Justice Drug Facts," 2020; Christine Vestal, "New Momentum for Addiction Treatment Behind Bars," *Stateline*, April 4, 2018, https://stateline.org/2018/04/04/new-momentum-for -addiction-treatment-behind-bars/; Christine Vestal, "This State Has Figured Out How to Treat Drug-Addicted Inmates," *Stateline*, February 26, 2020, https://stateline.org/2020/02/26/this-state-has-figured-out-how-to-treat -drug-addicted-inmates/; W. Sawyer and P. Wagner, "Mass Incarceration: The Whole Pie," Prison Policy Initiative, 2024, https://www.prisonpolicy.org/reports /pie2024.html, accessed November 1, 2024.

24. I. A. Binswanger et al., "Mortality After Prison Release: Opioid Overdose and Other Causes of Death, Risk Factors, and Time Trends from 1999 to 2009,"

Annals of Internal Medicine 159 (2013): 592–600, doi: 10.7326/0003-4819-159 -9-201311050-00005; E. L. C. Merrall et al., "Meta-Analysis of Drug-Related Deaths Soon After Release from Prison," *Addiction* 105 (2010): 1545–54, doi: 10.1111/j.1360-0443.2010.02990.x; C. J. Mumola, J. C. Karberg, and Bureau of Justice Statistics, *Drug Use and Dependence, State and Federal Prisoners, 2004* (US Department of Justice, Office of Justice Programs, 2007); S. I. Ranapurwala et al., "Opioid Overdose Mortality Among Former North Carolina Inmates: 2000–2015," *American Journal of Public Health* 108, no. 9 (2018): 1207–13.

25. J. G. Clarke et al., "The First Comprehensive Program for Opioid Use Disorder in a US Statewide Correctional System," *American Journal of Public Health* 108, no. 10 (2018): 1323–25, doi: 10.2105/AJPH.2018.304666.

26. Disaster Center, "District of Columbia Crime Rates 1960–2019," https://www.disastercenter.com/crime/dccrime.htm, accessed August 31, 2024; Robert DuPont, interview "Drug Wars," *Frontline*, PBS, https://www.pbs.org /wgbh/pages/frontline/shows/drugs/interviews/dupont.html, accessed May 1, 2021; R. DuPont and M. Greene, "The Dynamics of a Heroin Addiction Epidemic," *Science* 181, no. 24 (August 1973): 716–22, https://cdn.nixonlibrary.org /01/wp-content/uploads/2018/10/22130830/37-The-Dynamics-of-a-Heroin -Addiction-Epidemic-1.pdf.

27. DuPont, interview.

28. Donfeld, interview.

29. Baum, *Smoke and Mirrors*, 44; Donfeld, interview.

30. Jaffe, interview.

31. Baum, *Smoke and Mirrors*, 44.

32. Richard Nixon Foundation, "President Nixon Declares Drug Abuse 'Public Enemy Number One,'" April 29, 2016, https://www.youtube.com/watch?v =y8TGLLQlD9M.

33. Baum, *Smoke and Mirrors*, 56.

34. Norman E. Zinberg, "The Crisis in Methadone Maintenance," *New England Journal of Medicine* 296 (1977): 1000–1002, doi: 10.1056/NEJM197704 282961714.

35. Jaffe, interview; German Lopez, "Was Nixon's War on Drugs a Racially Motivated Crusade? It's a Bit More Complicated," *Vox*, March 29, 2016, https:// www.vox.com/2016/3/29/11325750/nixon-war-on-drugs.

CHAPTER 11: THE FALL

1. Marie Nyswander, interview with David Courtwright, June 22, 1981.

2. Jerome Jaffe, interview with Melody Glenn, June 15, 2021; M. Nyswander, interview.

3. Jaffe, interview.

4. Institute of Medicine (US) Committee on Federal Regulation of Methadone Treatment, *Federal Regulation of Methadone Treatment*, ed. R. A. Rettig and A. Yarmolinsky (National Academies Press, 1995), PMID: 25121195.

5. Stuart Auerbach, "Babies Born Addicted to Methadone: Methadone Causes New-Born Addicts," *Washington Post*, February 26, 1972; Kirk Scharfenberg, "Methadone Overdose Kills Youth: Methadone Overdose Kills

D.C. Youth, 18," *Washington Post*, August 18, 1973; Ron Shaffer, "Patient in Methadone Line Is Shot Dead: Methadone Patient Slain," *Washington Post*, July 11, 1972.

6. M. Nyswander, interview.

7. William L. Claiborne, "Methadone Hearings Set By Fauntroy: Fauntroy Schedules Methadone Hearing," *Washington Post*, October 11, 1972.

8. Zoe Adams, "The Nixon-Era Roots of Today's Opioid Crisis," *Washington Post*, April 20, 2023.

9. Michelle Alexander, *The New Jim Crow: Mass Incarceration in the Age of Colorblindness* (New Press, 2010), 55.

10. Robert DuPont, interview with Melody Glenn, June 23, 2021.

11. Charles Winick, interview with David Courtwright, January 25, 1993.

12. Santi Holley, "How Acupuncture Became a Radical Remedy in the Bronx," *Atlas Obscura*, https://www.atlasobscura.com/articles/lincoln-detox -radical-roots-acupuncture, accessed December 13, 2021.

13. Brynn Holland, "The 'Father of Modern Gynecology' Performed Shocking Experiments on Enslaved Women," *History*, December 4, 2018, https://www .history.com/news/the-father-of-modern-gynecology-performed-shocking -experiments-on-slaves.

14. Robert Baker et al., "African American Physicians and Organized Medicine, 1846–1968: Origins of a Racial Divide," *JAMA* 300 (2008): 306–13, doi: 10.1001/jama.300.3.306.

15. Austin Frakt, "Bad Medicine: The Harm That Comes from Racism," *New York Times*, January 13, 2020, https://www.nytimes.com/2020/01/13/upshot /bad-medicine-the-harm-that-comes-from-racism.html.

16. Richard Severo, "Rumor, Intrigue, and Criticism Beset City's Brooklyn Methadone Center," *New York Times*, June 11, 1970.

17. Beny J. Primm, *The Healer: A Doctor's Crusade Against Addiction and AIDS* (Create Space Independent Publishing Platform, 2014).

18. Institute of Medicine (US) Committee on Federal Regulation of Methadone Treatment, *Federal Regulation of Methadone Treatment*.

19. Institute of Medicine (US) Committee on Federal Regulation of Methadone Treatment, *Federal Regulation of Methadone Treatment*.

20. Institute of Medicine (US) Committee on Federal Regulation of Methadone Treatment, *Federal Regulation of Methadone Treatment*.

21. Institute of Medicine (US) Committee on Federal Regulation of Methadone Treatment, *Federal Regulation of Methadone Treatment*.

22. S. K. Rubel et al., "Scope of, Motivations for, and Outcomes Associated with Buprenorphine Diversion in the United States: A Scoping Review," *Substance Use & Misuse* 58, no. 5 (2023): 685–97, doi: 10.1080/10826084.2023 .2177972.

23. Z. Adams et al., "Changes in the Provision of Take-Home Methadone for People with Opioid Use Disorder During the COVID-19 Pandemic: Implications for Future Policymaking," Florida International University Legal Studies Research Paper No. 22-17, in *COVID-19 and the Law: Disruption, Impact, and Legacy*, ed. I. Glenn Cohen, Abbe R. Gluck, Katherine L. Kraschel, and Carmel

Shachar (Cambridge: Cambridge University Press, 2022), https://ssrn.com/abstract=4276877.

24. L. A. Goldsamt et al., "The Impact of COVID-19 on Opioid Treatment Programs in the United States," *Drug and Alcohol Dependence* 228 (2021): 109049, doi: 10.1016/j.drugalcdep.2021.109049.

25. S. Brothers et al., "Changes in Methadone Program Practices and Fatal Methadone Overdose Rates in Connecticut During COVID-19," *Journal of Substance Abuse Treatment* 131 (2021): 108449, doi: 10.1016/j.jsat.2021.108449.

26. C. M. Jones et al., "Methadone-Involved Overdose Deaths in the US Before and After Federal Policy Changes Expanding Take-Home Methadone Doses from Opioid Treatment Programs," *JAMA Psychiatry* 79, no. 9 (2022): 932–34, doi: 10.1001/jamapsychiatry.2022.1776.

27. Health and Human Services Department, "Medications for the Treatment of Opioid Use Disorder," *Federal Register*, February 2, 2024, https://www.federalregister.gov/documents/2024/02/02/2024-01693/medications-for-the-treatment-of-opioid-use-disorder.

28. Rubel et al., "Scope of, Motivations for, and Outcomes Associated with Buprenorphine Diversion in the United States."

29. Jaffe, interview.

30. "Title 21—Food and Drugs," *Federal Register* 37, no. 242 (December 15, 1972), https://www.govinfo.gov/content/pkg/FR-1972-12-15/pdf/FR-1972-12-15.pdf#page=90.

31. J. H. Jaffe and C. O'Keeffe, "From Morphine Clinics to Buprenorphine: Regulating Opioid Agonist Treatment of Addiction in the United States," *Drug and Alcohol Dependence* 70, no. 2 Suppl. (May 21, 2003): S3–11, doi: 10.1016/s0376-8716(03)00055-3.

32. Jaffe and O'Keeffe, "From Morphine Clinics to Buprenorphine."

33. V. P. Dole, "Hazards of Process Regulations: The Example of Methadone Maintenance," *JAMA* 267 (1992): 2234–35.

34. M. Nyswander, interview.

35. SAMHSA, *Federal Guidelines for Opioid Treatment Programs*, January 2015, https://store.samhsa.gov/sites/default/files/d7/priv/pep15-fedguideotp.pdf, accessed November 1, 2024.

36. M. Nyswander, interview.

37. MOTAA (Modernizing Opioid Treatment Act).

38. H. L. F. Cooper et al., "When Prescribing Isn't Enough: Pharmacy-Level Barriers to Buprenorphine Access," *New England Journal of Medicine* 383, no. 8 (August 20, 2020): 703–5, doi: 10.1056/NEJMp2002908. .

39. L. G. Hill Cooper et al., "Perceptions, Policies, and Practices Related to Dispensing Buprenorphine for Opioid Use Disorder: A National Survey of Community-Based Pharmacists," *Journal of the American Pharmacists Association* 63, no. 1 (January–February 2023): 252–60, doi: 10.1016/j.japh.2022.08.017; Larry Houch, "Prescribing Red Flags and Suspicious Controlled Substance Orders: Current Cautionary Tales," *FDA Law Blog*, December 5, 2023, https://www.thefdalawblog.com/2023/12/prescribing-red-flags-and-suspicious-controlled-substance-orders-current-cautionary-tales/.

40. Dan Baum, *Smoke and Mirrors: The War on Drugs and the Politics of Failure* (Little, Brown, 1996).

41. Jaffe, interview.

42. Alexander, *The New Jim Crow*, 49.

43. W. J. Bukoski, "Drug Abuse Prevention Funding Resulting from the Omnibus Budget Reconciliation Act of 1981," *Journal of Drug Education* 16, no. 1 (1986): 51–55, https://doi.org/10.2190/XUWW-YVUA-URJB-PPKN.

44. Maia Szalavitz, *Undoing Drugs: How Harm Reduction Is Changing the Future of Drugs and Addiction* (Hachette, 2021), 116.

45. Szalavitz, *Undoing Drugs*.

46. Alexander, *The New Jim Crow*, 54.

47. Alexander, *The New Jim Crow*, 55.

48. Szalavitz, *Undoing Drugs*.

49. Alexander, *The New Jim Crow*, 53.

50. W. Sawyer and P. Wagner, "Mass Incarceration: The Whole Pie," Prison Policy Initiative, 2024, https://www.prisonpolicy.org/reports/pie2024.html, accessed November 1, 2024.

51. Sawyer and Wagner, "Mass Incarceration."

52. Sawyer and Wagner, "Mass Incarceration."

53. ACLU, "Fight for Smart Justice," https://www.aclu.org/issues/smart-justice/mass-incarceration, accessed August 31, 2024.

54. Paul Brodeur, interview with Melody Glenn, June 24, 2021.

CHAPTER 12: UNANSWERED QUESTIONS

1. Paul Brodeur, interview with Melody Glenn, June 24, 2021.

2. Matthew Kassel, "Homo Correctus: Paul Brodeur Sues 'American Hustle' to Set the Record Straight," *Observer*, November 11, 2014, https://observer.com/2014/11/homo-correctus-paul-brodeur-sues-american-hustle-to-set-the-record-straight/.

3. Kassel, "Homo Correctus."

4. Harrison Smith, "Paul Brodeur, Journalist Who Exposed Asbestos Hazards, Dies at 92," *Washington Post*, August 10, 2023, https://www.washingtonpost.com/obituaries/2023/08/10/paul-brodeur-dead/.

5. Leonard Robinson, interview with David Courtwright, February 26, 1992.

6. K. Meehan et al., *Banned in the USA: The Mounting Pressure to Censor*, PEN America, September 1, 2023, https://pen.org/report/book-bans-pressure-to-censor/.

7. Joyce Lowinson, interview with Melody Glenn, May 15, 2021.

8. Marie Nyswander Robinson, *The Power of Sexual Surrender* (Chicago: Phocion Publishing, 2019), Kindle ed.

9. Robinson, *The Power of Sexual Surrender*.

10. Associated Press, "Women ARE Different from Men!," *Plain Dealer*, May 15, 1962.

11. David Courtwright, interview with Melody Glenn, March 15, 2021.

12. Patricia Goedicke to Pat Green, July 15, 1968, Patricia Goedicke and Leonard Wallace Robinson Papers, Series III: Correspondence, 1926–2006, University of Montana-Missoula, Mansfield Library, Book 31.

13. Dorothy Nyswander, interview with David Courtwright, February 17, 1992.

14. Steve Almond, "Introduction," in Cheryl Strayed, *Tiny Beautiful Things: Advice on Love and Life from Dear Sugar* (Knopf, 2012), https://www.penguin randomhouse.ca/books/217211/tiny-beautiful-things-by-cheryl-strayed /9780307949325/excerpt.

CHAPTER 13: GRASSROOTS

1. Robert DuPont, interview "Drug Wars," *Frontline*, PBS, https://www.pbs. org/wgbh/pages/frontline/shows/drugs/interviews/dupont.html, accessed May 1, 2021.

2. Associated Press, "From Rep. John Lewis, Quotes in a Long Life of Activism," *Washington Post*, July 18, 2020, https://www.washingtonpost.com/national /from-rep-john-lewis-quotes-in-a-long-life-of-activism/2020/07/18/7ee684d8 -c8b0-11ea-a825-8722004e4150_story.html.

3. SAMHSA, Center for Behavioral Health Statistics and Quality, *National Survey on Drug Use and Health (NSDUH)*, 2015.

4. S. Gutwinski et al., "The Prevalence of Mental Disorders Among Homeless People in High-Income Countries: An Updated Systematic Review and Meta-Regression Analysis," *PLoS Medicine* 18, no. 8 (2021): e1003750, doi: 10.1371/journal.pmed.1003750.

5. B. R. O'Shaughnessy et al., "The Recovery Experiences of Homeless Service Users with Substance Use Disorder: A Systematic Review and Qualitative Meta-Synthesis," *International Journal of Drug Policy* 130, no. 104528 (August 2024), doi: 10.1016/j.drugpo.2024.104528.

6. C. Simon et al., "We Are the Researched, the Researchers, and the Discounted: The Experiences of Drug User Activists as Researchers," *International Journal of Drug Policy* (July 20, 2021): 103364, doi: 10.1016/j.drugpo.2021 .103364.

7. A New PATH et al. to Members of the 118th Congress, March 15, 2024, https://downloads.asam.org/sitefinity-production-blobs/docs/default-source /advocacy/letters-and-comments/methadone-resources/sign-on-letter-support -and-motaa---03.15.24---finalv2.pdf?sfvrsn=b10e0516_1.

8. Helen Redmond, "Did ASAM Fight to Limit Federal Methadone Reform Bill?" *Filter*, July 25, 2023, https://filtermag.org/asam-methadone-reform-bill/.

9. AATOD, "The Modernizing Opioid Treatment Access (MOTA) Act: Fact-Checking Sheet," June 2023, https://www.aatod.org/wp-content/uploads/2023 /06/MOTAA-Fact-Sheet_FINAL3.2023-1.pdf, accessed November 1, 2024.

10. A. H. Kral et al., "Evaluation of an Unsanctioned Safe Consumption Site in the United States," *New England Journal of Medicine* 383, no. 6 (August 6, 2020): 589–90, doi: 10.1056/NEJMc2015435.

11. I. Rammohan et al., "Overdose Mortality Incidence and Supervised Consumption Services in Toronto, Canada: An Ecological Study and Spatial Analysis," *Lancet Public Health* 9, no. 2 (February 2024): e79–e87, doi: 10.1016 /S2468-2667(23)00300-6.

INDEX

abstinence-based treatment, 5, 18,
61, 69, 78–79, 102–3, 112, 118,
123, 144, 147. *See also* addiction
medicine
acceptable harm concept, 104–5
"addict," as a term, ix. *See also*
people who use drugs (PWUD)
addiction: and allyship, 111–12; common medical complications, 15;
criminalizing of, 16–17, 69, 77–78,
82; dependence vs., 5; as a disease,
16, 18–19, 26; genetic factors, 16;
as hopeless, untreatable, 15, 66–67;
as a moral or spiritual failing, 16;
supply versus demand debate, 111;
trauma experiences and, 16. *See
also* substance use disorder
Addiction (journal), article about
Nyswander in, 25–26
addiction medicine: at Berle's
clinic in Harlem, 117–18; board
certification requirements, 1–2;
consult services, 128; dearth of
medical focus on, 15, 70; Dole's
joining field of, 132; focus on
marginalized communities, 32;
governmental regulation, 6, 8,
53, 128–29, 158–59; Herring's
commitment to, 46; hodgepodge
approaches to care and treatment,
15–16; impacts of the Harrison

Act, 67–68; Jaffe's role, 149;
limited medical school instruction
related to, 14–15; medical board
complaints, 60–61; psychiatric
perspectives, 32; and redemption narratives, 185; therapeutic
communities, 152–53; treatment
vs. harm reduction, 49, 58, 102–3,
186. *See also* harm reduction;
methadone maintenance pro-
grams; stigma
Addiction Research Center (ARC;
Narco), 80, 82–86, 133. *See also*
Narco (Lexington, Kentucky,
Narcotic Farm)
Addiction Services Agency (New
York City), 144
Alameda, California: Glenn's work
in, 72; Nyswander childhood in,
28–29
Albert Einstein Medical College, 144
Alcohol, Drug Abuse, and Mental
Health Services Block Grants, 163
Alexander, Michelle, 154
allyship, 111–12
Almond, Steve, 176–77
Althusser, Louis, 146
"AMA" (against medical advice)
discharges, 125, 141
American College of Academic Ad-
diction Medicine, 189